BirdFlu
What To Do

Verona Fonté, Ph.D., filmmaker, psychologist, peace activist, and now writer, saw a crucial unmet public health need and has moved to fill it. She makes an important contribution to people everywhere with this down-to-earth, detailed, and practical guide to dealing with an avian influenza or other viral pandemic, which will one day come. Each of us must face the facts and take personal responsibility. This book leads the way.

  –Ted Mohns, M.D.
  Associate Clinical Professor, UCSD School of Medicine

US citizens have had ample opportunity to see the weaknesses in government's response capabilities for hurricanes, floods, and other natural disasters. Verona Fonté has written an excellent guide to assist citizens to prepare for a pandemic. Her book, Bird Flu What To Do *is easily understandable and presents a comprehensive planning approach to pandemic preparation. Readers who follow through on her suggestions should have the ability to protect themselves, their family, their businesses, and their neighborhood from the hazards associated with an outbreak of a pandemic disease.*

  –Joshua Lichterman, Ph.D. in Contingency Planning for Disasters
  President of the Emergency Management Group, Inc.
  Management consultant to corporations in emergency
  preparations

This book is an excellent resource for any disaster, natural or human-made. We never know when one will hit—and preparedness is a number one priority to save not only your life, but also the lives of your family, friends and neighbors. Moreover, for infectious disease, a healthy immune system is our best protection, and, since it's compromised by stress, being prepared is a great immune support.

  –Hyla Cass M.D., Assistant Clinical Professor of Psychiatry,
  UCLA School of Medicine, author of *8 Weeks to Vibrant Health*

Bird Flu
What To Do
PREPARE TO SURVIVE

Verona Fonté, Ph.D.

WITH CONTRIBUTIONS FROM

Grattan Woodson, M.D., F.A.C.P.
Ted Mohns, M.D. • Joshua Lichterman, Ph.D.
Kathleen Johnson, M.S., R.D. • Joan Halifax, Ph.D.

Iris Arts Press & Digital Media
Berkeley, California

Substantial discounts on bulk quantities are available to corporations, professional associations, and other organizations. Custom editions can also be accommodated.

For information contact:

Iris Arts Press & Digital Media
1856 San Antonio Avenue
Berkeley, CA 94707

order@birdfluwhattodo.com

This manual is intended to provide general information, and is distributed with the understanding that the author is not engaging in rendering legal, medical, or other professional services, and is not to be construed as legal, medical, or technical advice.

Cover and book design by Jan Camp, www.jcampstudio.com

*Premiere Edition published by Iris Arts Press & Digital Media
with Fort Creativity Publishing*

Printed in The United States of America

Distributed by Chelsea Green Publishing

ISBN: 0-9771037-1-4

www.birdfluwhattodo.com

1 2 3 4 5 6 7 8 9 UNITED 10 09 08 07 06

To my children and grandchildren;
and to all the young ones in the world.
May we create a safer and more
sustainable world for them.

Contents

APPENDIX A – C

Preface

What a turbulent time we live in!

Just glance at a newspaper or turn on the television for a reminder of how vulnerable we are to natural disasters. In shock, we watched as disasters such as the tsunami in 2004, Hurricane Katrina in 2005, and the earthquake in Pakistan in 2005 overwhelmed helpless victims. We've been stunned and scandalized by images of people who lost loved ones and homes and have been cut off from assistance. No one is ever fully prepared for the horror of a calamity, but universal denial and lack of preparation expose people to more pain and devastation than necessary.

We've all had the thought: What would I do if such a disaster hit close to my home? Am I prepared to survive a major emergency? This book will help prepare you, your loved ones, and your community to survive a natural disaster like the bird flu.

I had my first wake-up call several years ago when a friend phoned to alert me to the Avian Flu (referred to as the bird flu or an influenza pandemic in this book). He spoke as a physician and a concerned citizen when he described in vivid detail how a bird flu pandemic could impact the world. We wondered why there was so little attention being focused on this issue at the time. When I began my research I, too, became alarmed, but when I began sharing the information with family and friends, the response I received was lukewarm; most didn't want to dwell on apocalyptic fantasies. My children rolled their eyes, heaved deep sighs, or just looked at me politely. Friends didn't ask follow-up questions, so I changed the subject. And still, the media was reporting little information about the bird flu.

As a psychologist I understand denial, the impulse to avoid uncomfortable feelings associated with confronting an unwanted situation. Nevertheless I felt alone. People assumed I was paranoid, but my interest was based in my belief that, to people who have a sense of mastery over a situation, the world seems like a safer and saner place. For my doctoral research I studied women going through an unexpected stressful life transition—divorce. I found that those with a sense of environmental mastery (those who believed they had the skills and means to take care of themselves) were both psychologically and physically healthier during and after a divorce than women who did not. When people believe they have the capacity to care for themselves, they react less fearfully to unexpected stress.

The more I learned about the bird flu, the more clearly I saw the makings of a disaster: take a potentially lethal and easily transmissible virus, add ignorance and a lack of preparation, and you have something to be frightened about. A typical reaction to fear is "fight or flight." You might have the impulse to take *flight*: pretend it isn't happening, escape to the country, or padlock your doors and take care of your own. Or you may be moved to *fight*: get a gun, take what you need, and protect yourself. Some will automatically rush to help others while some will have trouble taking care of themselves. When a catastrophe occurs, everyone will react differently.

So be prepared for diverse responses. One of the major challenges we face (in our families, neighborhoods, and societies) is learning how to communicate and work together despite our differences. During a natural disaster we will all have to practice listening, patience, and understanding until we have found a way to bridge our differences and prepare everyone to survive. It begins with your family. Recently my son gave me a hand-cranked radio for my birthday, a gift that pleased me doubly because it showed he was listening and reflected his willingness to engage in the conversation about disaster preparation.

After Hurricane Katrina (and the disaster after the disaster when the state and federal governments failed to provide adequate assistance), I asked myself, *what was the lesson here?* It's probable that basic services will be disrupted during a natural disaster. We ordinary citizens have to be ready. We have to accept the fact that on some level we're on our own.

In short, we must prepare to survive!

I believe...

- we all need to be prepared to feel safe.
- survival planning is the most socially responsible thing we can do.
- we cannot count on governments to take care of our needs during a disaster.
- unless everyone in a community is physically and psychologically prepared for disaster, we create opportunities for social injustice and chaos as many of the most vulnerable will be left to fend for themselves.
- we are all caring people who can work together to preserve our loved ones, our neighborhoods, and the fabric of our communities from disaster.
- communities, neighborhoods, and families that have made the effort to prepare to survive natural disasters will be more resilient if and when a natural disaster occurs.

Acknowledgments

So many people have helped and supported me in putting this book together: my family, friends, cohorts, editors, contributors, endorsers, and consultants. I feel blessed to have such an extensive and generous network of people in my life. First, I want to thank my friend Ted Mohns, M.D., who first suggested that I investigate the Avian Flu (following this with a year of communication about how this phenomenon was developing), for his ideas about and contribution to this book. I want to thank E.R. Anderson, M.D., for endorsing this book, and helping me to reach networks otherwise inaccessible. His confidence in this project has sustained me throughout the process. Deep thanks to Leonard Duhl, M.D., for his support throughout, suggestion about the format of the book, and endorsement. Much gratitude is owed to my book consultants: Jan Camp, book designer; Susan Fassberg of Connecting Dotz; along with Mark Kohut, in New York, in bringing this book to fruition. Also, thanks to my wonderful daughter-in-law, Anna Fonté, M.A., who is an incredible editor. Big thanks to Daniel Susott, M.D., for being on the other side of any request when I needed to check medical facts. And thanks to John Fewings, the cartoonist from Ontario, whose subtle humor graces this book. Deep appreciation must be expressed to Candace Ford, the head librarian at Planetree Library in San Jose, who has encouraged, supported and consulted with me throughout this process. And thanks to John Russell who stepped in and took over the technical aspects of the website: www.birdfluwhattodo.com.

I want to thank my contributors for their generosity, time and belief in this book: my sister, Joan Halifax, Ph.D., who both contributed to the book and was always there with words of encouragement; Gratton Woodson, M.D., for allowing me to use his excellent material on how to care for someone with the flu at home; Joshua Lichterman, Ph.D., for his confidence and contribution on how workplaces need to prepare to create both safety and continuity of business during emergencies; and Kathleen Johnson, M.S., for compressing the breath of her knowledge about nutrition into such a short space.

Gratitude is owed to the people not already mentioned who took the time to read this book, and then offered to endorse it because they saw it as a useful addition to the literature on this subject: Hyla Cass, M.D., contributed expertise to the section on strengthening one's immune system; and Daniel Ellsberg, Ph.D., who dedicated his entire life to creating a safer world and could see the connection between his work and the underlying premise of this book. I also want to thank Christina Shaheen, M.Sc., my Project Manager, for her incredible support, competence and intelligent guidance.

A big thanks to other consultants in different arenas who vetted sections of this book for me or connected me to people who could assist me: Emanuel Ramirez, head of Environmental Health for the City of Berkeley; Sergeant Mary Kusmiss from the Berkeley Police Department Community Service Bureau; Kathy Roy from the San Francisco Water Utilities Department; Suzi Goldmacher, R.N., and Claire Greensfelder, of the Martin Luther King Jr. Freedom Center, Oakland. And thanks to Margo Baldwin for believing in this project. Everyone mentioned has helped make the writing of this book possible, and I am deeply grateful to each person.

I also want to thank my good friends who have supported me with kindness and encouragement throughout this process: Patricia Ellsberg; Jan Camp; Sooz Fassberg; Lowell Brooks; Nicole Milner; Vivienne Verdon-Roe; Jim Pelkey; Patrice Wynne; and last but not least, Joan Marler and Dan Smith (with whom I had the conversation that moved me to write this book), and the entire staff at their incredible French restaurant in Berkeley, Le Theatre, who always met me with good cheer, and fed me when I was too tired to fix dinner. They were my home away from home.

Finally, I want to thank my children, Dana, John and Anna, and my grandchild, Kenyon, for their support and connection even as I've disappeared into the assignment of writing this book.

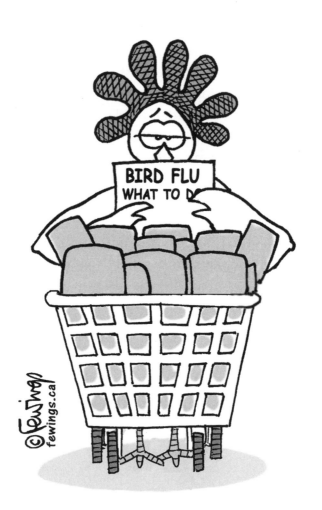

PREPARE TO SURVIVE:
THE BASIC NEEDS

→

Success depends upon previous preparation, and without
such preparation there is sure to be failure.
—Confucius

1.

Expect the Best—
Prepare for the Worst

NATURAL DISASTERS are any terrible event, not caused by human activity, which results in death, injury, or damage to property.

A PANDEMIC is a large-scale epidemic affecting a country, a continent, or the world that occurs when a new virus emerges in a population and spreads widely because people have not developed resistance to it and thus have little or no immunity, resulting in an unusually high number of illnesses and deaths.

THE BIRD FLU, also known as H5N1 influenza, is a new virus. Presently it is an avian disease and rarely affects humans. But health officials fear it will mutate into a form that can be passed easily from human to human, starting a pandemic in which millions of people may die.

It is difficult to start a book like this without invoking fear. But fear and grief would be natural reactions to a global pandemic. By taking the time to consider the scariest possibilities and then taking the appropriate precautions, you increase your chances of maintaining a sense of balance under emergency circumstances. Retaining sanity if chaos rules—that's the goal here!

If the bird flu hits your community and people get sick, the public systems we count on (hospital health care, mail delivery, public transportation, and normal delivery of goods) might falter. In a worst-case scenario, normal supply lines could be disrupted, creating a domino effect that would impact what goods are available. Quarantines could also impact the flow of goods, or transportation carriers could be re-routed elsewhere for emergency purposes. After Hurricane Katrina, refrigerator trucks were requisitioned to the New Orleans area, impacting deliveries elsewhere. If delivery of chlorine were disrupted, the water utility may not be able to deliver potable water to your home. Likewise, if supply lines were disrupted, this could impact the electrical grid. The invisible connections that keep everything running smoothly may become frayed. Social gatherings and public interactions would be discouraged to avoid contagion. Businesses could close. Unemployment would soar in areas that were hit the hardest. People might be asked or told to stay at home for their safety. Schools would shut down. We'd feel closed-in and stir crazy at home without work, school, or regular activities to distract us.

In hospitals, all the usual events will occur: children will be born, medical procedures will be performed, and people will have accidents and become critically ill. But in a pandemic, medical services will be besieged by the additional load of people with influenza, not to mention the other medical emergencies that will occur because of the scarcity of medicine, supplies, and equipment. Medical personnel will have to make difficult decisions about who gets attention. Police and emergency services will be stretched thin and personnel may be unable to respond to calls for help. Social disruption will occur if supplies are not available. Stores could be looted and home robbery may increase. Garbage may pile up, and stray or abandoned animals may rummage in it. We may have to take care of sick relatives. We may be approached by neighbors who haven't prepared for this crisis. While our municipalities begin to make plans about what to do if the bird flu becomes a reality, we might find that we're on our own. We all need to plan how to be self-sufficient and prepare to survive.

If there's a global influenza pandemic, professionals expect it will last a year or two, passing through communities in waves lasting several months. Everyone will be exposed to the virus: some will not be affected, some will get a mild case of the flu, some will survive more severe episodes, and some will not survive. If you survive an initial exposure to the virus, your body will develop varying degrees of immunity. However it is also possible for survivors to become reinfected if the virus modifies into a strain that isn't detected by the body's immune system.

No one knows for how long you need to prepare to be truly self-sufficient. For earthquakes and hurricanes, the rule of thumb is to have provisions for two weeks. I suggest planning to be self-sufficient for *at least* 30 days, assuming things would break down intermittently, get fixed, and then break down again. This proposal is not based on any objective data because there are none.

Plan for one month at least.
It's a mid-point between
crazy paranoia and dumb denial.

2.

Water Is Essential to Life

Water, water, everywhere, nor any drop to drink.
—Samuel Taylor Coleridge (1772–1834)

We cannot live without water. Loss of safe drinking water is deadly. Most individuals will begin to experience side effects from dehydration after 36 hours. There are many situations that may create a temporary interruption to the public water supply system: impassable highways, quarantines, and lack of equipment. If pipes are broken, no water can be delivered. Or if non-potable groundwater or sewage infiltrates into the water pipes, your water utility company may issue a "boil water" order or "unsafe water" alert, which means your water must be treated before you use it. Bottled water will quickly disappear from stores. Companies that deliver 5-gallon containers of water to homes and businesses will run out of stock.

Water storage for a pandemic is different than for other emergencies. Water storage is not necessary until a pandemic has reached your region, so your preparation is to have water storage containers on hand. You want to fill the containers with tap water when a pandemic is moving into your region.

How Much is Enough?

I suggest stockpiling at *least* one month's worth of emergency supplies per person. In an emergency situation, each person needs at least two gallons of water a day for the basic necessities (drinking, cleaning, and cooking). If someone in your household gets ill they will need to drink even more water each day.

Plan to have at least 60 gallons of water for a month's supply for every family member.

10 days = 20 gallons of water per person

20 days = 40 gallons of water per person

30 days = 60 gallons of water per person

60 days = 120 gallons of water per person

How Do I Store It?

All the containers listed below are safe for the storage of water. This means that unsafe chemicals from the containers won't leach into the water. The collapsible containers are obviously preferable for small homes or apartments that have little storage space.

- A 55-gallon water storage container with a siphon pump. This is not portable, but holds almost a month's worth of water for one person.

- A Nitro-Pack 20-gallon is a portable container.

- A 25-gallon Boxed Water Kit has five 5-gallon boxes that are collapsible for storage purposes. This system uses Mylar bags, which discourage the growth of microorganisms.

- A 5-gallon collapsible container such as a Reliance container.

- A 7-gallon rigid Reliance container, which is also small enough to be portable.

- Local water delivery companies may deliver 5-gallon containers already filled with water.

- Glass containers: water can also be stored in glass containers, but glass containers can break.

These containers may be available locally in hardware or camping stores. They can also be purchased online. For sources and websites, see page 112 of Appendix A in the back of this book and my website at *http://www.birdfluwhattodo.com.*

Water that is stored for emergency situations should be changed every six months to ensure the water supply continues to be safe. After a period of time microorganisms may start to grow in stored water containers, making it unsafe for drinking. Rotate store-bought water as well as water you've treated yourself. Store water in a cool, dark place. If you don't have such a storage space, change stored waters more frequently, (say every 3 months) to ensure it's safe to drink. Ingesting water containing microorganisms can cause a wide variety of illnesses depending on how it was contaminated, ranging from mild gastro-intestinal distress to serious disease such as typhoid and hepatitis.

All storage containers, (except for the Boxed Water Kits, which use Mylar bags), should be cleaned thoroughly before use. Wash with soap and water, rinse thoroughly with water, and then rinse again with a solution of water and a little chlorine before storing.

How Do I Make Sure It's Okay to Drink?

During an emergency, if there is any question about the purity of the water, treat it all before using it for drinking, food preparation, or hygiene. Chlorine (in the form of *sodium hypochlorite*) is used to treat over 95% of US tap water. Boiling, purification tablets, and water purifiers are commonly used to purify water during emergencies and outdoor activities.

Boiling is the safest method of purifying water, but it requires fuel. Boil water for 3 minutes.

Purification tablets release chlorine or iodine. They are inexpensive and available at most sporting goods stores and some drugstores. Follow the package directions. Usually one tablet is enough for one quart of water.

Water purifiers are devices through which you filter your water. They are different and more effective than *micro filters* or *water filters*. If a water filtration system is how you choose to purify your water, be sure you use a water purifier.

Chlorination[1] is used to purify water.

Water storage purification using chlorine (household bleach)

For storage, tap water should be purified in thoroughly cleaned plastic water storage containers to prevent the growth of microorganisms. Use a regular Clorox type bleach containing 4% to 6% sodium hypochlorite.

Do not use scented bleach or bleach with sodium hydroxide in it.

Water should smell and taste like chlorine, or it is not purified. If it doesn't, add a little more bleach until you can smell or taste it. Then stir and let stand for 30 minutes. Let particles settle to the bottom or strain them through layers of paper towel or clean cloth. Seal your water containers tightly and store them in a cool, dark place away from the sun to discourage the growth of microorganisms. This level of treatment will kill bacteria and viruses and prevent the growth of microorganisms for up to six months.

FOR PURIFYING WATER & SANITIZING SOLUTION
USE Sodium Hypochlorite
DO NOT USE Sodium Hydroxide

The following are guidelines for purifying water with household bleach:[2]

2 drops of bleach	per	1 quart of water
8 drops of bleach	per	1 gallon of water
1/2 teaspoon of bleach	per	5 gallons of water
1 teaspoons of bleach	per	10 gallons of water

Where Else Can I Get It?

You **must** purify water that comes from these alternative sources:

- Your bathtub (fill it if you think the water will be cut off)
- Rainwater
- Rivers
- Lakes
- Natural springs

- Ice cubes

- Water pipes

- Reservoir tank of the toilet (not the toilet bowl)

- Water heater

  o Before you drain your water heater, turn off the electricity or gas for the water heater by unplugging it or turning off the gas valve.

  o Open the drain at the bottom of the tank.

  o Start draining water by turning off the water intake valve and turning on any hot water faucet.

  o Do NOT turn on the gas or electricity for the water heater when the tank is empty.[3]

Do NOT use water from toilet bowls, waterbeds, radiators, or swimming pools/spas.[4]

→ **Water Preparation at a Minimum**

Get containers for water.

Have bleach in your home.

3.
Food Basics: What To Get and How To Store It

Contributed by Kathleen Johnson, M.S., R.D.

If you have the food you need, you'll feel more secure.

How Do I Store It?

- When buying food, choose only those that satisfy the nutritional and emotional needs of your family. Store food they like to eat.

- Slowly build up the non-perishable food in your house until you have enough for 30 to 90 days. Mark the date of purchase on the containers and use the oldest items first.

- Check food carefully and regularly for spoilage. Eat stored food before it expires and replenish the supply.

- Store food in a dry, cool place. The lower the temperature, the longer the shelf life.

- Containers should be clean and insect-proof with tight-fitting lids. Choose metal or plastic containers. Glass containers are safe but breakable.

- When storing food in plastic containers, use only those made for food. (Other plastics, including garbage bags, are not safe for food as they may be coated with chemicals that can leach into your food.)

- Store food off the floor (raise with boards or solid material if necessary), and away from cleaning supplies and other household chemicals.

- Buy freeze-dried, dehydrated, canned or regular dry staples.

- Foods that are freeze-dried and nitrogen-packed in cans have the longest shelf life and are more compact for storage. They are also the most expensive.

- Dehydrated foods won't last as long as freeze-dried foods, but can be vacuum-packed for long shelf life.

- Canned foods have a long shelf life, but are heavy and bulky. Keep some high-water canned foods like tomato products or fruits. Avoid jars when possible because they can break.

- Regular dry staples (like rice and noodles) generally require energy/fuel to prepare. Don't rely on them completely.

You need to have at least one BALANCED MEAL *and* TWO QUARTS OF WATER *a day to maintain energy and normal body functions. A variety of foods is best.*

What Goods Should I Get?

Vegetables

- Freeze-dried vegetables are available in stores and via the internet.

- Dehydrated vegetables need to be stored carefully to prevent spoilage.

- Canned vegetables such as tomato products can be useful because they are full of liquids.

Grains and grain products

Store these carefully in containers with tight-fitting lids to avoid infestation of weevils or other insects. Remember, the oil in whole grains increases the chance of rancidity or staleness.

- Wheat, rice, quinoa, oats

- Crackers (they keep longer than bread)

- Pasta

- Ready-to-eat cereals and hot cereals

- Flour and corn meal (white flour stores the longest)

Legumes

Store uncooked beans, dehydrated beans, lentils, or split peas. Combine legumes with grain when serving for a complex, full protein. This is important if there is a meat shortage.

Dairy

Milk is a good source of protein and calcium.

- Dry milk powder is available in whole, nonfat, or buttermilk versions.

- Aseptically packaged or "boxed" milk does not need refrigeration and has a shelf life of 6 months.

- Canned milk is another alternative.

- Aseptically packed soy beverage is also available. Choose a calcium-fortified version. Rice milk is mostly a carbohydrate and does not have the protein of dairy milk or soy beverage.

Other protein sources

- Freeze-dried or dehydrated meat and chicken
- Jerky or dried meat
- Canned fish such as tuna, salmon, or sardines
- Dried egg powder
- Nuts (store in closed containers to avoid staleness)
- Peanut butter

Fruits

- Dried fruits such as apricots, raisins, and apples need to be stored in sealed containers (preferably vacuum-sealed) to avoid spoilage. Store in a cool place.

- Freeze-dried applesauce powder is available.

- Canned fruits are useful to have as they contain liquids.

Fresh food that can be kept up to a few months if stored in a cool dry place

These can be kept up to a few months if stored in a cool dry place

- Onions
- Potatoes
- Yams
- Turnips
- Carrots
- Lemons
- Garlic
- Sweet potatoes
- Beets
- Chili peppers
- Sprouts
- Apples, fresh or dried

Comfort foods and little extras

- Honey, sugar, or canned syrup for a sweetener
- Oil, canola or olive
- Hard candy
- Chocolate bars
- Freeze-dried coffee
- Tea bags
- Instant hot chocolate mix
- Nuts

> DO NOT *underestimate the importance of comfort food during an emergency. The smell of coffee, for example, or the aftertaste of chocolate, can make everything feel almost normal.*

Tidbits

• If electrical power is disrupted, avoid opening and closing the refrigerator or freezer door. Use perishables as soon as possible and discard spoiled items. Eat the food in your refrigerator first, then the food in your freezer.

• Consider buying a flour grinder and a bread machine.

• Supplement your diet with a basic multivitamin and mineral supplement.

• If you have a pet, don't forget pet food.

• The U.S. Food and Drug Administration (FDA) states that no one has been infected with the bird flu virus by eating poultry or eggs that are properly cooked (165 degrees Fahrenheit or 74 degrees Celsius). Avoid eating or tasting foods that may contain raw or lightly-cooked eggs.[1]

(Refer to Appendix C, on page 128, for further recommendations about what foods to store.)

→ Food Preparation at a Minimum

**Begin to slowly build up
your non-perishable food at home now.**

Check expiration dates regularly and replenish the stocks.

4.
When the Lights Go Out

Equipment Considerations

During a power outage, unplug all electronic equipment, including televisions, radios, computers, washer, and dryer: this will lighten the load on the power system when electricity comes on. If you keep at least one light on you will know when the power is turned on. If your neighbor's power is on but yours is not, you have probably blown a fuse. Learn how to change or switch your fuses if you don't already know how.

Learn Where Your Utility Valves Are and How to Turn Them Off

Know where the electric, gas, and water shut-off valves are in your home and know how to shut these off. Knowing how to turn off the incoming water valve to your home is important in emergencies for the following reason: if there are reports of broken water or sewage lines, you need to shut off the incoming water valve to stop contaminated water from entering your home. Have the necessary wrenches to do the job and keep them near the gas and water shut-off valves in case there is damage to your home or you are instructed to turn off utilities. Teach family members how to shut off these valves. If you don't know how, ask a neighbor, call your utility company, or inquire at your hardware store.

If you turn the gas off, a professional must turn it back on.

Do not attempt to do this yourself. All pilot lights need to be relit and if this is not done properly there is a risk that natural gas may build up to a dangerous level which could cause an explosion, a fire, or asphyxiation.

KEEP SOME CASH ON HAND!
Large and small bills as well as loose change. If there is no electricity, banks will close and the ATM won't work.

Useful equipment to consider

- Matches: Books or boxes. Don't store all matches in one place.
- Candles, preferably long-lasting ones.
- Liquid paraffin is candle wax in liquid form at room temperature. It is both odorless and smokeless and is extremely safe to burn. A quart provides approximately 200 hours of candlelight and costs about $10. It is available at most camping and garden supply stores or online.
- Extra batteries: back up quantities for all battery-operated devices you have.
- Extra oil and wicks for lanterns.
- Extra fuses (for old-fashioned electrical systems).
- L.E.D flashlights: not expensive and longer lasting than regular flashlight batteries.

- Some stores sell a L.E.D. flashlight that fits on your head. Petzl has one that lasts 150 hours at low setting, 80 hours at a high setting.

- Long-distance L.E.D. flashlight.

- Hand-generated flashlight.

- Battery charger: solar-powered or with a hand-crank.

- Propane canisters and kerosene that fit your cooking/heating equipment.

- Hand-cranked or battery-operated radio.

- Gasoline generator: expensive but worth it.

Cooking without Power

There are many alternatives, just make sure you've planned ahead and have one in place.

- Camp fire or fire pit.

- Outdoor barbecue grill.

- Coleman stove (use propane canisters).

- Esbit Pocket Stove: this is an emergency stove used by the military. It's a short-term solution; the heat source is a tablet so you would need a stock of tablets.

- The Trangia Minitrangia 28-T Stove uses denatured (drug store) alcohol[1] as a heat source.

- Nuwick candles are nontoxic paraffin candles that are used for light, heat, and cooking. They use removable, reuseable wicks, and you can increase the light and heat output by using more than one wick. You can buy them at most camping supply stores or online.

- The folding stove that uses Nuwick candles.

- Extra briquettes.

- Propane tank(s) for outdoor grills.

- Extra tanks and canisters for the type of cooking device that you have.

(In Appendix C, on pages 132–133, you will find the tear-out list of power supplies, cooking supplies, and solar suggestions.)

→ Power Outage Survival, at a Minimum

Know how to turn off all utilities.

Have flashlights, candles, and batteries.

Have an alternative way to cook.

5.
Sanitation Sanity

There are things you never thought you'd want to learn.
Some of them are in this chapter.

Clean Kitchen, Clean Cooking

- In case of a bird flu pandemic, keep the food preparation area clean to avoid contamination. The virus can be carried into the house on the bottom of bags, on the paws of your pets, or on your shoes. Leave shoes at the door.

- Clean all food preparation surfaces with a sanitizing solution of 1 teaspoon of household bleach (5.25% sodium hypochlorite, Clorox type bleach) in one gallon of water. Follow these steps: Wash with soap and water, rinse with water, clean with sanitizing solution, and then let dry.

- For rinsing dishes and utensils, use a sanitizing solution of 1 teaspoon of household bleach per gallon of water. If you are washing dishes with cold water, use a solution of 1 tablespoon of bleach for each gallon of water. Allow dishes to soak for 10 minutes. You can reuse this sanitizing solution throughout the day.

- Always wash your hands in hot soapy water after you have handled raw meat, poultry, or fish. Always avoid contact between raw and ready-to-eat food. Use a separate cutting board for raw food and fresh food, and never put fresh or cooked food on a plate that previously had raw meat, poultry, or fish.

Important: The Center for Disease Control recommends discarding wooden cutting boards, baby bottle nipples, and pacifiers because they cannot be properly sanitized.

SANITIZING SOLUTION FOR CLEANING
1 teaspoon household bleach per 1 gallon of water.

RINSING SOLUTION FOR WASHING DISHES IN COLD WATER
1 tablespoon household bleach per 1 gallon of water.

Toilet Trouble

That's right: if the water system does not work, neither do the toilets!

When your toilets are not working you need to know how to create makeshift toilet facilities for health and convenience. This means creating the toilet and making sure human waste is securely contained so animals and insects have no access to it (as they can spread disease). When possible, **separate liquid from solid waste**. This decreases the volume of the human waste, allows it to dry more quickly, and makes it easier to store if there are delays in disposal.

- After using any makeshift toilet, cover waste with baking soda or lime *(calcium carbonate)*, which you can get from a hardware store. This is non-toxic, prevents the growth of pathogens, dries the waste (making it easier to handle and store), and helps control the odor.

- Flies breed in solid waste so keep latrines tightly covered to avoid unsanitary conditions and the spread of disease.

Makeshift Toilet Facilities

Example 1

Use your toilet. If the water is not working, after you flush the last water out, the toilet bowl will be empty. At this point turn off the water valve behind the toilet to ensure that water does not flow into the toilet bowl in case the water system is turned on while you are using it for a makeshift toilet. Clean your empty toilet with a household bleach like Clorox and water. Line the toilet with two heavy-duty plastic garbage bags. Cover the toilet tightly after use to keep flies and pests away. (You will need a cover that will prevent insects from entering the toilet.) As stated above, separating human waste from liquid is recommended, so try to urinate in a separate container and dispose of this down a drain or on the ground outside.

Example 2

Use a 5-gallon plastic bucket fitted with a toilet seat. These can be purchased as a ready-made unit, or you can make your own by putting a toilet seat on top of a 5-gallon bucket. Line with two heavy-duty plastic garbage bags. Cover toilet tightly when not in use to keep flies and pests away.

Example 3

If you don't have an extra plastic bucket available, you can make a latrine by digging a long trench approximately one foot wide and 12 to 36 inches deep. Each time you use the latrine, cover your waste with lime or baking soda and then 12 inches of soil. When you dig a latrine too deep it can slow the bacterial breakdown process, so don't dig it deeper than 36 inches. Avoid contaminating potential water sources by placing the trench more than 100 feet away from any water source. The location of the latrine should also be away from your living area and where animals won't disturb it. Mark the site so others know what is buried there and in case the city later wants to properly dispose of waste for health reasons.

We take our basic conveniences for granted.

How to Dispose of Waste

Your local environmental health department will probably have a solution to the problem of solid human waste disposal if the water utilities are disrupted. Ask them about this now to encourage them to think about this issue.

They may:

• send trucks to neighborhoods for waste collection.

• have you dump waste in an operating sewer located in your neighborhood.

• place chemical toilets in neighborhoods.

- ask you to bury your waste material (in a pit 12 to 36 inches deep, covering it with 12 inches of soil, as explained in Example 3).

But if your city has no plan to set in motion, it's important that you have ideas about temporary disposal methods for solid human waste:

- Dig your own latrine as described above in example 3.

- Deposit solid waste in a working sewer line in your neighborhood that remains sealed tight when not in use.

- Tightly seal your bags of waste and put them in a secure place away from your living space and inaccessible to animals until the local environmental health department gives you further instructions.

Garbage and Rubbish

Garbage is waste that will spoil or decay, such as leftover food (e.g. compost).

Rubbish is waste that will not spoil or decay, such as paper and glass products (e.g. recycling material).

- Separate the garbage from the rubbish. Compost your garbage if you can.

- If you can't compost, put garbage in plastic bags that you tie tightly when full, and place in a watertight container. If garbage collection is not going to happen within 10 days, ask your environmental health officials what to do or find a way to bury garbage. If garbage is not tightly sealed it becomes a breeding ground for flies. Information about how and where to dispose of garbage should be available from local environmental health officials.

- People living in apartments and in dense urban neighborhoods should request information from their city about what to do with garbage before a crisis occurs.

- Keep animals away from buried waste and garbage because if it's contaminated they may spread the virus.

- Sickroom waste could be infectious and should be handled carefully and separately from regular garbage. It should be double-bagged, sealed tightly, and stored away from locations where animals have access to it until regular pickups are available.

- Rubbish disposal is not as critical as garbage disposal and rubbish can be stored in open areas.

- Depending on local fire regulations you can burn combustible rubbish such as cardboard and paper for heat if necessary.

→ Sanitation, at a Minimum

Have bleach.
Have heavy-duty plastic garbage bags.
Buy baking soda or lime *(calcium carbonate).*

6.
Keep Your ID—
Keep Your Records

Although it's not who we are,
many of these documents become our "official" identity.

Keep copies of important family records in a waterproof, portable container for emergencies. Having these documents available after a disaster enables you to restore normal life more quickly. You will immediately be able to contact important people in your life and access your health insurance, bank accounts, and other assets and public records that are important to you.

Wills • insurance policies • contracts • deeds • stocks and bonds • passports • driver's license • social security cards • immunization records • durable power of attorney • living will • bank account numbers • credit card account numbers and companies • inventory of valuable household goods • important telephone numbers • family records (birth, marriage, death certificates)

Refer to Appendix C, page 134, for an extensive list of documents you want to consider having handy.

→ **IDs and Records, at a Minimum**

Passport

Driver's License

Bank And Credit Cards

Telephone Numbers

7.
Healthy Habits

Keep Your Germs to Yourself

*Washing and drying your hands
is the most important way to protect yourself
against the spread of germs.*

Washing Hands

Wash hands with soap and warm water for 20 seconds or more
or use antiseptic hand wash.

- After washing, thoroughly dry hands, preferably using disposable tissues or towels. If you have a virus on your hands, by using a disposable towel you eliminate the chances of spreading it to someone else.

- You can clean hands with an alcohol-based hand sanitizer, which kills both bacteria and viruses. These are available at local grocery and drug stores.

*When to wash hands?
Simple answer: almost all the time!*

Wash Hands

- After shaking someone's hand.

- Before preparing food.

- Before eating.

- After coughing.

- After touching surfaces in public places such as doorknobs, tables, handgrips.

- After touching money.

- After using the toilet.

- When caring for sick persons.

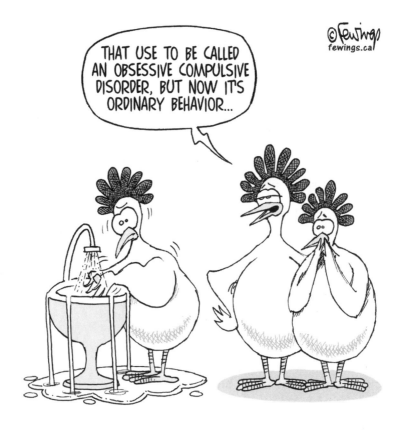

STOP Hand-To-Face Contact

Change this habit now. We unconsciously touch our face all the time. Be aware of this pattern and each time you notice you are touching your face try to remember to stop it. Every time we bring our hand to our face, we bring whatever germs and viruses are on our hands to our face, increasing the chance of infection.

• We prop our head up with our hand.

• We scratch our chin.

• We wipe our mouth.

• We rub our nose.

Everyone Should Practice the Following Cough/Sneeze Etiquette:

• Keep your mouth and nose covered when coughing.

• Coughing or sneezing into the crook of one's arm will limit the spread of germs.

• Use disposable tissue and immediately dispose of the tissue.

• After coughing, wash and dry hands thoroughly.

• Avoid close contact with other people if you are sick.

• If you are sick or coughing and are around people, you may want to wear a N95[1] mask to avoid contaminating them. Use masks to protect yourself and to protect others. (See page 36, under "Pandemic Fashions: Masks and Gloves," for detailed instructions.)

Teach your children these habits now.

Viruses can be transmitted for approximately two days before a person is showing any symptoms and for at least a week after symptoms have disappeared.

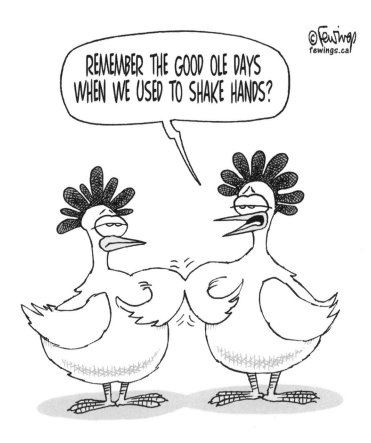

You never know when you're being exposed to a virus.

Social Distancing During a Pandemic

If there is a bird flu pandemic or any kind of infectious disease outbreak, social distancing will become a popular concept. To avoid catching the flu if there is a pandemic, we must:

- Minimize contact with others.

- Stop attending large gatherings and going to public places such as the movies.

- Try to maintain a safe distance (about a yard or a meter) between people when possible.

- Try to hold neighborhood meetings in open spaces where you can maintain a safe distance between people.

- Remind people who are ill that they should isolate themselves as much as possible.

- Remind those who are ill to use a disposable N95 mask to help prevent exposing others to the virus. The mask should be carefully disposed of after it becomes moist or after any cough or sneeze. Then hands must be thoroughly washed and dried.

- Put a QUARANTINE sign on your front door or on your lawn to alert others if someone in your home is sick.

These behaviors are crucial to slowing
the spread of the bird flu if there is a pandemic

Pandemic Fashions: Masks and Gloves

Personal protection equipment includes N95 masks, goggles, eye/face shields, gloves, gowns, and aprons. Nothing fancy, but for home use consider masks and gloves. They can be purchased at a drugstore. Disposable N95 masks are "must haves" when:

- People are ill and want to protect others from their germs. If you only have one mask, it should be placed on the sick individual.

- You are caring for someone who is sick and want to try to gain some protection from their germs.

- Waste materials have to be handled.

The recommended N95 mask is made by various manufacturers under different names. For proper functioning, the N95 mask must fit securely to your face. Find the size that fits your face. The mask should have a metal clip that you bend over your nose. If there are gaps around the mask you can use tape

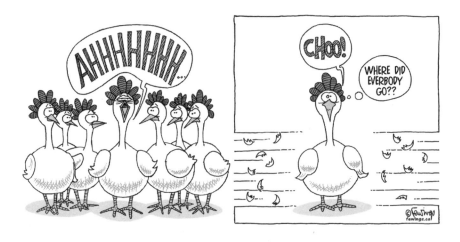

to secure it tightly. It should be thrown away if it becomes wet, if it interferes with breathing, or if it is damaged or soiled. If it has been exposed to a possible carrier of the virus, it is contaminated and should be thrown away. When discarding it, wash your hands prior to handling the mask. Remove it using the straps and throw away with other sick room materials. Wash your hands before and immediately after handling the mask.

Disposable gloves are useful when . . .

- taking care of someone who has the virus.
- waste materials have to be handled.
- cleaning up materials that may be contaminated.
- taking care of the body of someone who has died.
- handling money in public places.

Strengthen Immunity Now

- Get a vaccination against the flu each year. There is no vaccine for the bird flu, but you need to be vaccinated every year to help you resist the annual flu. If you catch the ordinary flu and the bird flu at the same time, your immune system will be overtaxed. In the U.S., vaccinations are free for people aged 65 years and over and for adults and children with certain long-term or chronic conditions.

- Eat a balanced diet with fresh fruits and vegetables.

- Take vitamins and minerals to supplement your diet. Talk to your health care provider about their recommendations.

- Drink at least 8 glasses of fluid daily.

- Consider vitamin C: In her book *8 Weeks to Vibrant Health,* Dr. Hyla Cass discusses natural ways to strengthen your immune system, highlighting the importance of Vitamin C.[2]

    o Under stress (like a viral infection), your need for Vitamin C increases.

    o When your body has had enough, you will experience soft stools or diarrhea, a sign that you have reached "bowel tolerance" (e.g. it is time to begin to lower the amount of vitamin C you are taking).

    o Once you start experiencing soft stools (it can be at 1 gram or 20 grams: your body will tell you), cut back to 25% of that dose and keep taking that dose daily. For example, if 20 grams of vitamin C gave you soft stools or diarrhea, you would then cut back to 15 grams.

    o Adjust that dose as needed in response to your body's signals (e.g. if you have loose stools, your dose of vitamin C is too high).

- Elderberry is often recommended to help fight influenza. There is an excellent critique of the use of elderberry on *http://www.fluwiki.com,* citing recent research and discussing potential advantages and problems with the use of elderberry products to strengthen the immune system in relationship to a bird flu pandemic.

- Stay in good shape psychologically. Learn how to manage your emotions so you can stay calm and feel more balanced during times of stress.

  o Shift your attention when you find yourself thinking about things that upset or scare you.

  o Practice paying attention to what you are doing in the moment. By developing this habit of focusing your attention you can learn to work with your emotions during difficult times.

  o Talk to friends when you need to express your concerns.

- Stay in good shape physically and maintain an exercise regime.

For additional information about strengthening your immune system, and alternative and integral health perspectives, go to our website at ***www.birdfluwhattodo.com***.

→ Healthy Habits, at a Minimum

Have a supply of gloves, N95 masks, antiseptic soap, and Vitamin C.

Wash your hands frequently, especially before and after contact with an ill person.

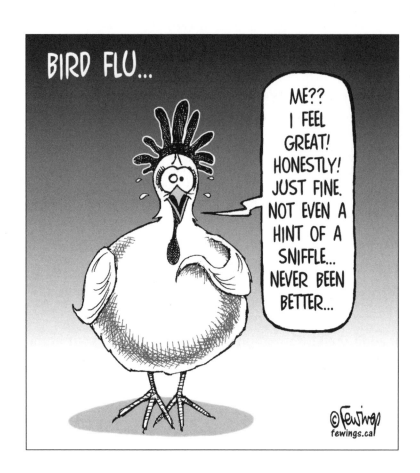

CREATE A SAFE
COMMUNITY

→

*How the community is organized, how people relate, what
institutions are involved, and how they collaborate is of utmost
importance in preparing to survive a natural disaster.*
—Leonard Duhl, M.D., F.A.C.P: Professor Emeritus,
University of California, Berkeley School of Public Health

8.
Building and Strengthening Your Support System

So far we've focused on preparation for individuals or households. Next we reach out to extended family, friends, and neighbors. Encourage them to prepare. Disaster preparation works best when we involve as many people as possible. If well organized, neighborhoods and communities are more resilient during disasters. Share this guidebook and your preparation strategy with others.

Be a Good Neighbor

- Call a neighborhood meeting. (See agenda ideas below.)

- Before the meeting, review your city's preparation plan. Look up the city/town's website or call city officials and ask what information is available about disaster planning.

- Review your state's plan at:
  http://www.pandemicflu.gov/plan/stateplans.html

- The purpose of the meeting is to encourage neighbors to start their own survival planning and to organize a neighborhood preparedness group.

- Brainstorm about how you can work together, what resources and expertise you can share, how you will communicate, and how you can take care of each other if there is a pandemic or other natural disaster.

Neighborhood Meeting Agenda Ideas

What knowledge do you need in an emergency, and what skills do people have? Among your neighbors you may find people with medical training, individuals with organizational, technical and maintenance skills, extraverts who like to keep up with what's going on with others in the neighborhood, cooks, etc. Discuss what skills people have and what responsibilities they can take on. Here's a list of suggestions:

The Neighborhood Communicator is the person who keeps track of what everyone in the neighborhood is doing. His or her role is to check in and see if anyone has special needs. (This can also be the person who encourages all neighbors to get involved in planning and preparation before an emergency occurs.)

Information Central keeps contact with other parts of the community and other neighborhoods after a disaster to learn the latest developments. This person stays in the neighborhood (if there is a quarantine) and receives and sends out important information. This should be someone who has a ham radio, walkie-talkie, or crank/battery-operated radio.

The Liaison makes physical contact with other groups and local governments to see what coordination is being developed. This person would leave the neighborhood and attend meetings with other groups during the emergency situation.

The Tech/Maintenance Person is someone who has basic maintenance and technical skills. This person can assist and consult with neighbors about how and when to turn utilities on and off, how to fix things, how to get equipment running again, etc.

Person(s) with medical, Community Emergency Response Team (CERT), or Cardio-Pulmonary Resuscitation (CPR) training can offer support. This person would be the consultant on neighborhood medical supplies, encouraging everyone to have their own medical kit, defining what should be in it, and also noting special equipment that is obtainable and can be potentially shared. This person would know where someone should go if they become ill. They would take responsibility for sharing information about end-of-life measures.

Cooks can volunteer to make sure food is delivered to all who are ill or don't have the energy to feed themselves. Also, if the neighborhood decides to buy food supplies in bulk, the cooks can organize the purchase and distribution of goods.

A Neighborhood Runner is a person who will take responsibility for spreading news in the neighborhood and for maintaining the neighborhood bulletin board.

Some of these roles can rotate among different people. This list is not complete nor comprehensive. You may have other ideas about roles and responsibilities in your neighborhood. The basic idea is to take advantage of the local resources and to share responsibilities in a way that benefits everyone.

What RESOURCES are there in the neighborhood that can be shared in an emergency?

- Recreation vehicles usually have their own generators, which would prove useful if electrical power goes down
- Generators
- Ham radios

- Walkie-talkies
- Bull horns
- Shovels
- Ladders, saws, other common tools, etc.
- Solar devices
- A well
- Extra food
- A swimming pool that can provide a source for water to wash with. DO NOT use water from a swimming pool for drinking water or cooking.

Meetings and Communication During a Quarantine

- Choose a meeting place for emergency situations, **preferably outside,** that can be used as a staging area. This is the place where all will meet when any natural disaster occurs to assess the damage and ascertain who needs help. (In an infectious disease situation, such as the bird flu, it is preferable to have meetings in the open so neighbors can maintain a safe distance to avoid infection.)

- Have a phone and email list of everyone in the neighborhood. Agree on other safe ways to communicate if electricity goes out or cell phones aren't working.

- Decide where you will place the neighborhood bulletin board.

Special Needs

Discuss how to encourage everyone in the neighborhood to create a survival plan.

- Try to understand the obstacles to full participation. Is it time, money, interest, or mobility? Find creative ways to include everyone.

- Continue to give people who are not involved all of the information you have.

- Make a list of neighbors with special needs: the elderly, people who live alone, the handicapped, and people who may be ill.

  o Find out what their plans are, what networks they have, and what assistance they need.

  o Make sure they are prepared for a disaster or contact family or friends that will take care of them in an emergency.

  o Make decisions about how the neighborhood can assist them.

  o Find out what resources are available in the community for people with special needs.

Special Situations

- Discuss openly what will happen if there is an emergency where food and water is in short supply and there are neighbors who have not prepared.

o One solution is to ask all neighbors to store extra provisions in case there are neighbors who have not stockpiled necessities, or to collect donations for people who may not be able to create a stockpile for themselves.

- Get information from your city about their plans for emergency provisions.

- Should a bird flu pandemic occur, agree on what people will do if they become sick.

  o Encourage people who become ill to self-isolate as much as possible in order not to infect others.

  o Strongly encourage people to practice healthy behaviors. (Review Chapter 7, "Healthy Habits," page 31.)

- If someone lives alone and becomes too sick to care for him- or herself, have a plan in place about what neighbors will do.

- Encourage all neighbors to have a designated "sick room" in their house with all provisions (medicines and protective equipment). This room should be as close to toilet facilities as possible. (In Appendix C, page 131, you will find recommendations for a home pharmacy. Also review Chapter 14, "If You Have To Play Doctor" on pages 86–87 regarding supplies to have in the sick room.)

- If the emergency lasts longer than expected, and the social fabric begins to unravel or violence comes into your neighborhood, how will the neighborhood and the community handle this situation?

  o Expect a wide range of responses. Some people will have weapons and feel that this is a time to use them. Others will believe this approach can only create more violence. (Refer to Chapter 12, "Protecting Your Turf and Staying Safe," page 67, for more information about this issue.)

o It is important to listen to each other, discuss differences, and find ways to cooperate and support each other in these situations.

o Discuss how you, as neighbors, will deal with and work through differences or conflicts.

o A crisis provides opportunities to respectfully work together despite differences.

Engage Your Community

Find out who in your city is in charge of disaster planning. Contact that person and ask them the details of their emergency disaster plan, and specifically what plans are in place if there is a bird flu pandemic.

Questions and Issues to Explore with City Officials

Stay Informed

• If communication systems are down, how can you know about important plans and developments in your community and how can you learn how to get needed resources?

• Are there emergency radio stations that would continue to operate even if the electrical grid is not working? Where are these stations and is this information being communicated to the community?

Disruption of Services

- What plans are being made about water storage and water dispersal if these services are disrupted?

- If garbage pick-up is disrupted, what will people be instructed to do? (The issue of garbage disposal poses a different situation if you live in an apartment building or a densely populated urban area, so find out what to do before an emergency occurs.)

Shortages

- Do the local food banks have enough supplies to handle a quarantine situation if normal food delivery is interrupted? If they don't and are not working with America's Second Harvest: The Nation's Food Bank Network, suggest they call this organization at 800-771-2303.

- How is your city coordinating essential commodity delivery (food, essential supplies, etc.) and rationing if the emergency lasts a long time and supply lines are disrupted?

- How will availability of essential commodities and drop-off points be communicated during an emergency?

- To mitigate social unrest due to a critical lack of supplies, will the city coordinate with local businesses to distribute supplies?

Medical Services

- How will the medical system operate if it is overwhelmed?

- How will the availability of medical services be communicated during a disaster?

- What will happen if deaths occur at home and the infrastructure to deal with the deceased is overloaded?

Working with All Socioeconomic Groups

- Are plans being made that take into consideration all socioeconomic groups?

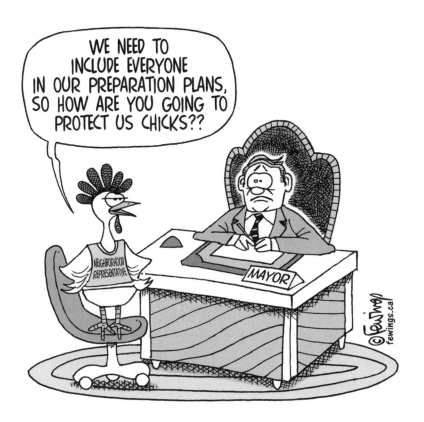

- Can individuals and groups with more financial means help support preparation efforts in lower-income areas in your community before there is an emergency?

- Can contributions be made to local food banks? If so, how or where can donations be made?

- What else can be done?

Safety and Security

- What is the role of police and fire personnel in a natural disaster?

- What are the plans if there is social unrest?

- Is your city council satisfied that adjacent cities are prepared to the extent that if there are shortages of food or water, there will not be spillover of need or violence into your city?

Other Actions and Behaviors that Will Be Useful Before and During an Emergency

- Bridge all socioeconomic groups in your planning.

- Find ways to encourage everyone in the community to prepare.

- Find ways your community, neighborhood, or church can start a fund to help lower-income neighborhoods prepare.

- Bartering: be creative about sharing and bartering both goods and services.

- Store extra food and supplies to either barter with or give to people who have not prepared as well as you have.

→ **Creating a Safe Community, at a Minimum**

**Find one or several people in your neighborhood
who will take charge of this effort.**

**Have a neighborhood meeting to discuss the issues that may
arise in an emergency situation like a bird flu pandemic.**

**Meet with local officials to address their
preparations for emergency procedures.**

9.
Workplace Preparation

Contributed by Joshua Lichterman, Ph.D.

"[A human outbreak of bird flu in the United States] is a 675 billion hit (in 2006 dollars) to the U.S. economy."
—U.S. Senate Majority Leader Bill Frist [1]

It's hard for one person to make a difference in the workplace in the case of a bird flu pandemic, but if management is open to survival preparation, here's what they should be thinking about. Show this section to your employer, and suggest that they craft a plan if they don't already have one. A worldwide pandemic would have a major impact on the ability of all organizations to continue "business as usual."

Whether the bird flu becomes a pandemic, it's both practical and far-sighted for all businesses, (large, medium, and small), to determine their ability to maintain operations by evaluating their vulnerability to disasters and developing a plan for the business to function despite a disaster (e.g. "a business continuity plan"). Organizations, like people, need to prepare to survive.

The first step in this effort is to identify the organization's points of vulnerability in the event of a natural disaster. Some of the issues addressed might be:

- Is the business tourism-related?

- Would the business suffer if people stayed away from shopping malls, restaurants, theaters, public transportation, etc.?

- How dependent are employees and customers on mass transit systems?

- Are the products or services considered vital for the national interest?

- What are the consequences of supply chain interruptions? In a pandemic, these breaks in the normal flow of goods will be due to inspection and logistics disruptions, particularly when the suppliers are in areas with high infection rates.

- Are there alternative means of transporting finished products?

Once it's understood how the organization would be effected by a natural disaster, a plan can be developed to support the continuation of business if there is a bird flu pandemic. This "business continuity plan" will include elements such as:

- Notifying employees about the bird flu threat and plans being made to continue to operate if there is a pandemic.

- Determining how to minimize its impact on the business:

    o Determining the minimum number of employees required to maintain the flow of products or services.

    o Establishing the ability to provide shelter and food for these skeleton crews.

    o Developing plans to allow the maximum number of

employees to telecommute and teleconference and securing the necessary hardware and software to make this possible. This may require changes in current corporate rules.

o Creating notification systems to allow management to communicate with all staff at work, at home, and in between to keep them informed of the changing situation.

o Generating notification procedures for informing customers, clients, shareholders, and the public about the state of the business—open, closed, limited production, shortages expected, etc.

o Expanding online transaction and self-service options for customers and vendors.

Finally businesses will need to decide how to best minimize the health emergency for staff, their families, and perhaps some of the general public who reside close to the corporate facilities. Protecting workers/contractors and their families helps ensure business continuation by attending to preparation efforts at the early stages. In this way, the business also gets the benefit of being recognized and appreciated for taking care of its corporate family. Some of the elements of such a prevention plan would include:

• Having a set of rules for employees, contractors, and visitors regarding when it is appropriate to come to work and when it is a disciplinary offense to come to work if someone is infected with the flu.

- Developing the ability to provide antibiotics or vaccines to all employees, contractors, and perhaps families and the general public living in close proximity to your facilities.

- Deciding whether to stockpile drugs/vaccines or to rely on public sector supplies and delivery systems.

- Deciding whether your plan is self-contained or in partnership with your county public health organization.

- Creating checklists that allow staff to provide emergency services to employees for a 6-10 day or a 48-hour scenario.

- Have annual trainings and exercises so that the staff is adequately prepared and ready to respond.

Many businesses have suffered in the recent past from natural disasters because they did not plan ahead of time, and some have never reopened their doors. Businesses have this choice as we face the coming pandemic: Take their chances, do nothing, and risk major negative impact, or be prudent, develop the necessary plans to be able to decrease the impact of a natural disaster, and recover quickly afterwards.

> → **Work Place Preparation, at a Minimum:**
>
> **Talk to your employers about their plans.**
>
> **If they have no plans, give them this book and refer them to an Emergency Management consultant.[2]**

10.
Communication

When there's a crisis, we want information and reassurance and we often get it over the phone. But telephone and cell phone services may be disrupted if there is a global pandemic. If the power grid goes down, you won't be able to recharge your cell phone (unless you have a battery/hand cranked radio-cell phone chargers or a generator). Service from maintenance crews can also be delayed if many people are sick and off work. During a natural disaster, the priority will be to maintain service to the government, police, fire stations, and hospitals. In other words, the personal needs of regular citizens will have to wait.

With Your Family

- If family members live in other locations, have a communication plan. Discuss what you will do if you are unable to communicate with each other by phone.

- Be prepared to have some silences if you live far away from each other.

- Revive letter-writing if postal services are operating.

- Use email if you can, but remember most email communication is by phone lines.

Reassure each other that. . .

- you have a survival plan in place and will take care of yourself in an emergency.

- you have a supportive network in your community.

- when the opportunity arises, you will try to communicate.

With Neighbors

- Have a phone and email list including everyone in your neighborhood.

- Have an agreed-on bulletin board location for the neighborhood.

- Have a way to communicate with other neighborhoods when phone services are not working, for example, with a neighborhood "runner."

With the Outside World

- It is important to have a battery-operated or a hand-cranked radio so you can get information about the status of the situation from whatever channels are broadcasting in your area.

- Find out what local emergency radio stations will be operating.

Ask you health care providers now, before a disaster, how you will be able to communicate with them if things get tough and communication through normal channels is interrupted.

Imagine a world without cell phones.

→ **Communication Preparation, at a Minimum:**

Have a phone and email list including everyone in your neighborhood.

Be prepared to survive without communication resources.

Have a battery-operated radio.

11.
Housebound and Stir Crazy

Contributed by Ted Mohns, M.D.

If a pandemic reaches your town or city and if you have chosen to stay where you are rather than leave for a month or two, the prudent thing would be to remain indoors for at least the first few weeks to avoid exposure to the virus. During that time, close contact, even with friends and neighbors, may be unwise since you can't know whether they've been infected.

Being cooped up in a house for weeks may be more difficult than you think. We are profoundly social creatures and we're accustomed to full freedom of movement and access to our social network. Being confined for weeks (whether alone or in the company of others) may lead to severe stress that can worsen by not knowing what's going on "out there." And when stress is experienced over a sustained period of time, judgment, physical health, and the strength of the immune system are all affected. So if we can foresee the difficulty of being housebound and predict cabin fever ahead of time, the negative impact can be mitigated.

If you expect to be confined to your house for several weeks...

- It's critically important to designate a decision-maker at home. That role may rotate among different members of the household. Prolonged emergencies are NOT the place for a total democracy. The decision-maker will not be perfect, but it will be better than having no one in that role at all.

- Write out a daily schedule or routine and stick to it. It will help everyone feel as though they are contributing to the solution and working together. Assign specific duties (e.g. radio monitoring, cooking, cleaning, etc.). Retain discipline; we humans need a sense of structure.

- Exercise at a mild aerobic level for 15-20 minutes twice a day.

- Plan events or projects to relieve the monotony. This may be a good time to fix the leaky faucet, write, clean out the attic, or look at old photo albums.

- Find ways to laugh. Humor is especially priceless under conditions of severe and sustained stress.

- Consider keeping a daily journal. Writing experiences down has a way of helping us make sense of events and making emotions seem more manageable.

- Remind yourself repeatedly of things you have accomplished in the past and take pride in the things you're doing well now. Exercises in simple self-esteem are a potent offset to sustained stress and feelings of powerlessness.

- Stock games, books, puzzles, art supplies, and other creative ways to pass the time.

- Go to sleep and get up at regular hours. Avoid long daytime naps.

- Singing and dancing can be powerful stress-management methods.

- Being frightened and essentially trapped for a while can often trigger periodic irritability and even feelings of aggression. Expect these feelings to emerge and plan for them in advance. If you need to, hit a punching bag or a pillow to let off steam.

- Within the group, find daily ways to give and receive love. Never forget the power of a kind word or a loving touch.

In an already difficult situation, you'll want to minimize anything that may create more stress, including focusing excessively on your confinement. Try to look at it as an opportunity rather than an utter tragedy. Perhaps this is a chance to finally organize your CD collection, fix up an old car, write a novel, or bond with your family.

> → **Housebound Preparations, at a Minimum:**
>
> **Discuss with your household how you would spend your**
>
> **time and issues that might arise if there is a quarantine**

12.
Protecting Your Turf and Staying Safe

In the last few years we've come to understand that disasters do occur and that we should all have survival plans; we should not live in fear but be prepared to survive in case we're caught in harm's way. If a community is not prepared for a natural disaster such as the bird flu, its basic infrastructure could deteriorate, creating widespread social disruption.

Under conditions of extreme stress (real or perceived), some people become heroic or altruistic. But when people do not have basic needs such as water, food, and shelter, some will do things that are selfish, desperate, or violent. Some of these people will have weapons and might think they have the right to take what they need.

Think through what you will do if everything goes haywire and people start acting erratically. Discuss this with family, friends, and neighbors. Have a neighborhood plan in place so you can support and protect each other if thieves come into your neighborhood. (There is safety in numbers. A lone robber is less likely to confront a group. They will generally select a vulnerable target as a path of least resistance.)

Be prepared to encounter different opinions about how to deal with these situations. Some people keep weapons in their homes and others don't. Try to reach an agreement about how to safely protect yourselves. The more eyes and ears on the street, the better equipped neighborhoods and communities are to reduce crime and assist local police in the apprehension of criminals.

Hope for the best; prepare for the worst.

Below are suggestions for theft protection organized from passive to active strategies.

You Stay Home

Contact your local police department and ask them about their recommendations for protecting your family and neighborhood from robberies. Suggest the community start a program involving your entire community that addresses how to lessen crime if there is a natural disaster such as a pandemic.

How to Protect Yourself from Robbery During a Pandemic

• Have a phone and website list of local emergency services.

• Reinforce windows and doors:

   o Get double bolts on your doors and windows.

   o Folding security shutters can be bolted to the interior of the window frame and closed if necessary.

   o Security-type film, which is reasonably transparent, can be applied to windows and extends onto the window frame, providing fairly good resistance to simple window-smashing attempts.

o Doors need to be solid, not hollow-core, and should have deadbolt locks or even a heavy bar that can be placed across the door in two brackets.

o Have a peephole in your door so you can see who is outside.

o Do not open your door for anyone you don't know.

- Pay attention to strangers in the neighborhood, alerting other neighbors to unusual behavior and contacting authorities immediately.

- Store goods in several locations so if you are robbed you will not lose your entire stockpile.

- Keep a low profile. Don't make yourself a target. Go to bed when it's dark and do what needs doing during the day.

- If you don't own a dog, place a large dog dish outside your door. You can even get a recording of a large dog barking. (Remember, this may need to be battery-powered if the electricity goes out.)

- Put a "Quarantine" sign on your lawn or front door. This may deter would-be thieves.

- Make sure your neighborhood plan includes what to do if you or your neighbors are threatened.

o Include a way to signal others if you need help: phone, gongs, flags, bullhorns, etc.

o If you have several bullhorns in your neighborhood, work out a strategy where neighbors could call off would-be thieves from several locations, distracting and discouraging them from breaking into someone's home.

o Small directional air horns run off of compressed air and put out roughly 130 decibels. The noise can be quite painful and even disabling.

- If you are interested in a protection strategy that will deter, but not harm, an assailant, consider pepper spray. It can be useful against suspects who aim to attack you physically. Pepper spray can also be used if the suspect has a knife or stick. It is not encouraged if the suspect has a gun. Information can be found at *http://www.peppersafe.com/ pepperspray/ocpepperspray/*

You Head for the Hills

This is an option if you have friends or family who live in the country and who will welcome you for an extended period of time. There is no guarantee you will be safer in the country. If a pandemic is severe and there's a shortage of supplies, there is the possibility for social disruption in both the city and the country. But in the countryside there may be a garden, a natural well, and less exposure to the virus.

If this is the strategy you choose, consider your options and plan carefully beforehand:

- Arrange this trip ahead of time. Know who is going, where you are going, and how you will get there. Have provisions in this location for at least 30 days per person or bring these provisions with you.

- Move *quickly* once it's apparent the crisis is going to occur because highways can become overwhelmed with traffic. Fuel could be in short supply and movement may become restricted if there is a quarantine situation.

- Make a checklist of everything you must do to safely close down your home.

- If possible, have a social network that plans to work together in your retreat location.

- Have a phone and website list of local emergency services in your new location.

Consider all of the security measures listed above under "You Stay Home."

One important note: If you are being robbed and someone has a gun pointed at you, do not struggle. Give them what they want. Usually thieves are as nervous as you are, and you don't want to do anything to escalate the situation.

→ Protecting Your Turf, at a Minimum

Decide whether you are going to stay home or head for the hills.

Contact local officials and consult with them about safety concerns.

Have a neighborhood and community plan for security issues.

SPECIAL NEEDS
AND SITUATIONS

→

Do unto others as you would have them do unto you

13.
Dependents' Needs

Children, the elderly, the disabled, and our pets need special consideration and help in any emergency. Plan for their well being.

The Kids

Talk with your children ahead of time about the reality of emergencies, describing possible scenarios.

- The Federal Emergency Management Agency website *www.fema.gov/kids* has good material to assist children in learning more about disaster preparedness.

Talk to your children's schools to find out their plan if there is a bird flu pandemic or quarantine in your community.

- Are your children being taught about disaster preparedness?

- Are children being taught about the importance of hygiene or healthy behaviors in school?

- Would home schooling be part of a plan if there is a bird flu pandemic, and if so, how would it work?

Consider the negative impact of repetitive or hysterical news coverage if a pandemic is predicted in your area and think about limiting children's exposure.

Issues to Discuss with Your Children

- Let your children participate as much as they are able in the family preparation strategy so that they feel they are in control. (Take them shopping, show them the phone list, etc.)

- Suggest they organize their own emergency kit and brainstorm together about what goes in it.

- What kinds of food would they like to have included on the family storage list, including "comfort food"?

- Discuss the possibility of staying home for an extended period. How would they see themselves spending their time? What would they like to amuse them at home? What activities might they enjoy that don't require electricity?

- Educate them about the importance of healthy behaviors such as hand washing, avoiding hand-to-face contact, and cough etiquette, and encourage them to start these practices now.

- Consider involving them in the neighborhood planning group and talking about what they would do during a period of isolation.

- Talk to your kids in a way that won't frighten them about what you will do if someone in the family gets sick.

Elders and Disabled

Those with special needs are the people who will need the most support during any natural disaster. These are family members, friends, or neighbors who are dependent on others.

Refer to the section entitled "People Who Can Help," page 80, for more information. Also, read the section about caring for the sick at home in Chapter 14, "If You Have To Play Doctor," on page 85. Take extra time to think about the needs of the elderly and disabled people in your life when you are making preparations to survive.

Who in your life or your neighborhood needs special assistance and how can you assist them with preparations?

- Do they have social networks in place?

- Do they have family members with whom they can live if there is a pandemic?

- If there are no support networks in place, what will the neighborhood do?

People with Special Medical Needs[1]

How to Survive a Disaster

In preparing for disaster, people with special medical needs have extra concerns. Try to picture yourself as you would be during such a disaster and during the period immediately following it. What are your needs and what do you need to do to survive for at least one month?

Emergency Bag

Have a bag packed at all times in the event you need to leave your home. In it include:

- A medication list and your medicines. Don't forget the ones in the refrigerator!

- At least a month's worth of medical supplies.

- A copy of vital medical records such as insurance cards, Living Will, Durable Power of Attorney, etc. (See page 134, in Appendix C for a complete list of records you may want to consider.)

Medications

- Always have an extra month's supply of all of your medications. Contact your health insurance company to make arrangements.

- Store your medications in one location in their original containers.

- Have a list of all of your medications: name of medication, dose, frequency, and the name and phone number of the doctor prescribing it.

Medical Supplies

If you use medical supplies such as bandages, colostomy bags, or syringes, have a supply available that would carry you through several months in case there is a disruption of supply lines.

Intravenous (IV) and Feeding Tube Equipment

- Know if your infusion pump has battery back-up and how long it would last in an emergency. Consider what arrangements or supplies you would need in a prolonged emergency.

- Ask your home care provider about manual infusion techniques in case of a power outage.

- Have written operating instructions attached to all equipment.

Oxygen and Breathing Equipment

- If you use oxygen, have an emergency supply. (The amount should be worked out with your health care provider.) Also check with your medical supply company to see that they are stockpiling extra oxygen tanks in case of a disruption of supply lines.

- Oxygen tanks should be securely braced so that they do not fall over. Check with your medical supply company regarding bracing instructions.

- If you use breathing equipment, have extra supplies of tubing, solutions, medications, etc.

- Discuss with your insurance company, your health care providers, and your community about how your special needs will be addressed in an extended emergency.

Electrically Powered Medical Equipment

- For all medical equipment requiring electrical power (such as beds, breathing equipment, or infusion pumps), check with your medical supply company and get information regarding a back-up power source, such as a battery or generator.

- Check with your local utility company to determine that back-up equipment is properly installed.

People Who Can Help

- An important part of being prepared to survive is planning with family, friends, and neighbors. Who could walk to your home to assist you? Who can bring you supplies if you need them? Who will look in on you if you're not feeling well?

- Discuss your disaster plans with your home healthcare provider.

- Does your local fire department keep a list of people with special medical needs?

- If you depend on electrical power for your medical equipment, notify your local power company. Some companies are able to provide priority service to people with special medical needs.

- Keep a list of people who can help, with their name and phone number:

    o Family or friends

    o Neighbors

    o Hospital

    o Medical suppliers

    o Doctor/homecare provider

    o Pharmacy

Don't Forget Your Pets

If you have a pet, undoubtedly they are part of your family and are dependent on you to take care of them in an emergency.

- If you decide to leave home and go to the country, take your pets with you.

- If you have dogs, it's important to keep them leashed and under your control as dogs can rummage through garbage, which might spread disease if there were a pandemic.

Stockpiling for Pets

You need to store both food and water for your pets for at least a month. Also you need to stockpile other supplies such as cat litter, litter box, leashes, medicine, etc.

Staying Informed

Stay informed about whether your pet is "at risk" of carrying bird flu and/or what to do for your pet if there is a pandemic. For more information contact The American Veterinary Medical Association's website with data and articles about bird flu and animals: *http://www.avma.org/*

Bird Flu in Cats: If there is a bird flu pandemic, the virus might spread to humans through cats. Cats that were fed raw infected poultry in Asia have developed bird flu. In January 2006, *The Journal of Pathology* reported in a study about cats and the bird flu that "pet cats might give people H5N1 after eating one of the many wild birds or poultry still infected across East Asia."[2] This means that if there are indications that the bird flu is in your region, pet cats must not be let out and they must not have contact with other cats or with wild birds that may be carrying the bird flu.

Bird Flu in Pet Birds: Pet birds need to be kept caged and not allowed to fly free where they might have contact with other birds that may be carrying the bird flu. It's important to keep their cages clean and to wash your hands thoroughly after you have contact with them.

> **→ Preparing for Dependents' Needs, at a Minimum**
>
> **Explore with your children what it means
> to have a natural disaster.**
>
> **Brainstorm what will entertain them while confined to home.**
>
> **Identify elders and people with special medical
> needs in your lives, and help them prepare.**
>
> **Prepare for your pets to survive.**

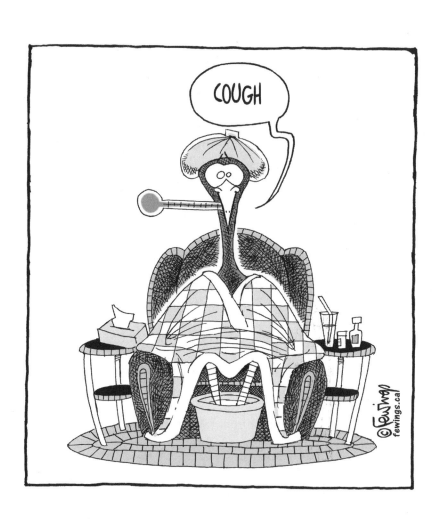

14.

If You Have To Play Doctor

Adapted by the Author from
"Good Home Care for Patients with Bird Flu"
by Grattan Woodson, M.D., F.A.C.P.

Treatment of Influenza at Home

Under the circumstances, having a supply of over-the-counter products and select prescription drugs on hand for the home treatment of cases of severe influenza is prudent. For instance, simple household items that will be very useful include ibuprofen, acetaminophen, table sugar, and table salt. It will also be helpful to have on hand, and know how to use, a thermometer, and an automatic blood pressure and pulse monitor. In the following discussion, I will provide you with advice on how these simple items can be used very effectively for the home care of flu sufferers. In order to obtain the prescription drugs needed for the home care of the flu, please call your doctor who is best able to advise you. I have included the over-the-counter and prescription items that I think will be most useful but your doctor may have other equally good or better suggestions especially since he or she knows your specific medical condition much better than anyone else. I call the medications, together with the household items, the "Flu Survival Kit."

Simple Medical Skills Required

Caregivers need to learn how to obtain vital signs like pulse, blood pressure, temperature and respiratory rate. It will also be very useful to be able to use an automated blood pressure monitor to measure blood pressure. These devices come with pretty good instructions that clearly explain how to use them. "Practice makes perfect" applies to learning and perfecting these skills. If you need help learning how to do these, ask your doctor or his/her nurse for help.

Prescription products for home treatment
of one person with severe influenza

- Tamiflu 75mg # 20: take two tablets daily for 5 (or 10) days for flu[1]

- Probenecid 500 mg #20 tablets: take 1 twice daily with Tamiflu

- Promethazine (Phenergan) 25mg tablets # 60: take ½ to 1 tablet every 4 hrs as needed for nausea

- Hydrocodone with acetaminophen (Lortab-5) # 60 (5mg/325mg): ½ to 1 tablet every 4 hrs as needed for cough or pain

- Diazepam (Valium) 5mg # 60: ½ to 1 tablet twice daily as needed for anxiety, muscle aches, or insomnia

Over the Counter (OTC) products to have on hand for
home treatment of one person with severe influenza

- Table salt: 1 lb

- Table sugar: 10 lbs

- Baking soda: 6 oz

- Household bleach 1 gal

- Tums Ex: 500 tablets

- Acetaminophen 500mg #100 tablets

- Ibuprofen 200mg # 100 tablets

- Caffeinated tea, dry loose: 1 lb

- Electronic thermometer: have two, in case one breaks

- Automatic blood pressure monitor: I recommend the hand pumped automatic BP monitor rather than ones with electric pumps.

- Notebook for recording vital signs and fluid intake and output

- Kitchen measuring cup with 500 cc (two cup) capacity

- Diphenhydramine (Benadryl) 25mg capsules # 60: 1 tablet every 4 hours as needed for nasal congestion, allergy, or itching.

Symptoms of Influenza

The influenza virus usually enters the body through the respiratory tract but can also gain access through the intestinal tract. The virus causes a variety of symptoms but the leading ones are fever, sore throat, cough, runny nose and general aches and pains. In addition to these principal symptoms, many also experience headache, nausea, abdominal cramps and diarrhea.

These symptoms could be due to some other infectious agent or even another strain of influenza virus since it is possible that both routine seasonal flu varieties and pandemic strains could be circulating in the community at the same time.

There are several ways to tell the difference between the flu and less severe illnesses. First of all, unless the flu is circulating in the community, then your illness is probably not the flu, because it tends to occur in epidemics that are easy to spot epidemiologically. If the world is in the midst of a major pandemic, you will have no problem knowing about it.

Also, the flu is much worse than simple cold viruses or most other causes of respiratory or gastrointestinal (GI) infections. The fever and body aches are really quite remarkable and often associated with strong shivering. Patients with flu are really sick and often are so weak that they have a hard time getting up out of bed without help. So, one way to tell the difference between the flu and other infections is that the flu is really severe and tends to affect the respiratory track most often, but can also cause severe gastroenteritis (nausea, vomiting, and diarrhea).

Patient Prognosis During Pandemic Influenza

One thing that is different about a major pandemic is just how hard it hits patients and how rapidly it kills. Patients affected by the flu can be broadly categorized into 3 prognostic types. The first type has a poor prognosis no matter what is done for them. The second might survive if there was full access to high technology medical care and resources. The third type is highly likely to recover from the flu as long as they are provided with consistent low-technology supportive measures that can be administered in home settings. (Refer to Appendix B, page 117 for a more thorough description of each type of patient.)

In my opinion, as a general rule, provide everyone with the same level of supportive care. This is a rational course because it is not always possible to predict who will survive and who will not, especially early in the course of the flu.

Using Scarce Resources Wisely

Patients in extremis, which means they are near death at the time they are encountered, should not be disturbed unless there is something that you can do to make them more comfortable. Fortunately, patients in extremis are usually already unconscious and beyond suffering.

If medical supplies are in short supply, especially those like the antiviral drug Tamiflu, the decision of how to ration these resources is best made by health professionals if they are available. If not, my suggestion is to concentrate your efforts and precious supplies on those with the best chance of survival. In a severe pandemic it is unwise to use limited medical resources on the critically ill, as they are unlikely to survive. So my advice is to focus your greatest efforts on patients where the prognosis is good for a complete recovery.

Preventing and treating dehydration in the flu patient will save more lives than all the other combined treatments

Supportive Treatment of Influenza

Home Flu Treatment Advice for Laypeople

Caring for severely ill flu patients is something that everyone is capable of doing. You can do this. No medical skill is required. The skills needed are the same that parents use to care for their young children or adult children use to care for their elderly parents. They need a soft place to lie down and they need to be comforted and told that they are going to be OK and reassured that you will be there for them. The most important medical treatment is to make sure they have plenty of fluids. Dehydration must be prevented, as this can be fatal in a patient who would otherwise survive.

> *The basic goals are to keep the patient*
> *clean, dry, warm, and well hydrated.*

Fever, Body Aches, Chills, Sore Throat, and Headache

Ibuprofen and similar medications, and/or acetaminophen are used to lower fever and help the patient feel better. The above symptoms respond well to these drugs. Use these products for the flu according to my instructions, not the bottle label. Don't under-dose the patient. Many people take doses that are ineffective for fear of taking too much. Remember that acetaminophen can be used at the same time as ibuprofen, both in full doses, because they are in different drug classes and have different drug side effects. Combination treatment with both has an additive effect of benefit without increasing risk. The dose of ibuprofen I recommend you use is 2 to 4 tablets (400mg to 800mg) every four hours. For the purposes of this guide, ibuprofen means aspirin, Advil, Aleve, ibuprofen, or Nuprin since they are all similar drugs. Acetaminophen (Tylenol) is in a different class of drugs than the ones just listed. For acetaminophen, the dose is two 500mg tablets 4 times daily. Do not exceed these doses for either drug. This is the maximum for both.

A very high fever (> 104 F) can cause seizures and brain damage and must be avoided. Using tepid water sponge baths works well for a high fever. Do not use alcohol sponge baths instead of water. Alcohol can be absorbed through the skin, especially in children, resulting in toxic effects. Ibuprofen and acetaminophen are very good at lowering temperature. Studies show that the body's natural defenses are better able to fight infection with some fever (say up to 101 F), so we shouldn't try to completely suppress the temperature to normal (98.6 F).

Gargling with hot salt water is a good treatment for sore throat. Hot caffeinated tea is also very helpful for headache, sore throat, and cough. We are taking advantage of the pharmacologic effect of caffeine, long recognized as an excellent herbal therapy for these problems. Hot or cold tea is also a mild stimulant that improves the sense of the patient's well being. Sore throats also respond well to ibuprofen or acetaminophen.

Food

Eating is not really important because the patient will be breaking down their own muscle and fat for energy. The flu takes your appetite away so the patient probably won't be hungry. If the patient is hungry and asks for food, this is great as it is a real sign of improvement. By all means feed the patient at that point but your food selection needs to be appropriate. Specific directions on how to feed patients recovering from severe flu are provided below.

Fluids

What will be much appreciated by a sick patient, especially if they are dehydrated, is a simple Oral Rehydration Solution (ORS) made from water, sugar and salt.

The Adult ORS formula "A" for dehydration
  1-quart clean water
  1 level tsp table salt
  4 tbsp table sugar

The Adult ORS formula "B" for dehydration due to diarrhea
  1-quart clean water
  ½ level tsp table salt
  ½ level tsp baking soda

The ORS formulas "A" and "B" treat dehydration caused by different symptoms of the flu. ORS "A" is an excellent treatment of dehydration due to sweating, decreased drinking, and vomiting. If the patient has become dehydrated because of diarrhea, use the alternative ORS "B" formula, because with diarrhea, patients lose bicarbonate that is replaced by the baking soda (sodium bicarbonate) in the formula. If they are both vomiting and have diarrhea, alternate ORS "A" with "B" to give a balanced therapy. This adjustment to the ORS will work very well.

Identifying Dehydration

Preventing dehydration in flu victims will save more lives than all the other treatments combined. When patients have a fever or diarrhea, they lose much more water from the body than is commonly appreciated. Symptoms of dehydration include weakness, headache, and fainting. Signs of dehydration include dryness of the mouth, decreased saliva, lack or very decreased urine that is dark and highly concentrated,[2] sunken eyes, loss of skin torpor (the elasticity of the skin), low blood pressure especially upon sitting up or rising from the sitting to the standing position, and tachycardia (fast pulse) when lying down or sitting up.

Fever is an especially easy way to become dehydrated with no one even noticing. That is because the loss of body fluid occurs through the skin and quickly evaporates. The smaller the body size and the higher the temperature, the faster this can happen. Water in the form of vapor is also lost through the breath. So, when the patient is short of breath and breathing rapidly, this is another source of hidden fluid loss.

If you detect or suspect that dehydration is developing, administer fluids by mouth. If the patient is too ill to drink, someone should sit with the patient giving him or her fluids drop by drop if needed. Work up to using a teaspoon if possible. Don't stop until the patient has been able to keep down at least a quart of fluids. This could take several hours so be patient. It will have a dramatic effect on a sick patient's well being. After the first quart, the patient should begin to urinate again. This is a good prognostic sign and when this happens you can assume you have restored their fluid level back to a safer level. "Safer" should not be confused with safe. Don't stop there. With sick patients like these, you really need to "push the fluids" so don't let your guard down.

This will be very refreshing for the patient and will quickly revive them. Fluids can be served cool or hot depending on the climate, patient symptoms, and fever status. A patient with a high fever should probably not be given hot fluids because it will raise his or her temperature further. A patient with a sore throat will get relief from a hot beverage. A patient hot with fever might prefer a cool or even cold beverage. If it is cold outside, especially if the patient is cold, use hot fluids. You can drink the ORS plain or flavor it with just about anything like citrus, mint, or herbs.

If juice is available, you can substitute 1 cup of it for 1 cup of the water and cut the sweetener in half. Administering fluids to the sick in your charge will be one of the main activities day in and day out until the crisis passes. Try to get 2 to 3 quarts of fluids down the patient every day at a minimum. Make this your most important task.

Preventing the Virus and Bacteria from Spreading within the Household

It is unlikely that we will be able to limit exposure to the virus if there are a lot of sick people around us. The flu is so easily passed from one person to the next that it is difficult to control even in the hospital setting.

In truth, pandemic influenza is so infectious that those of us taking care of sick folks in our homes are simply not going to be able to prevent being exposed to the virus. Even simply breathing the air in the vicinity of the sick will result in significant exposure. It is a fact we will have to accept.

Hand washing after coming into contact with the sick or with things that have been in contact with them is a very important method to avoid the spread of the virus or bacteria within the household. Use of a N95 mask may be effective in preventing the mask wearer from becoming exposed. It is most useful for preventing an ill person from spreading an infectious disease to someone else.

It will be very important to keep the sick and their bed and bed coverings clean and dry. Likewise, the sick rooms and bathrooms need to be maintained in good condition. The soiled garments and bedding will need to be washed and dried, a task likely to be made quite challenging if there is a lack of electrical and water service. It will be important to wash these soiled items in hot water using soap and chlorine bleach if possible. Hard surfaces should be wiped clean using soap and water and then sprayed with 1:10 bleach to water solution and wiped down a second time. This will effectively remove all trace of body fluids, vomit, and excrement and neutralize all infectious viral particles.

By recognizing the symptoms a patient has or the signs of the disease in the body, you can use the chart on the following pages to guide your treatment.

Caregivers and anyone in the vicinity of the sick, which will be virtually everyone, will be exposed repeatedly to the pandemic virus loads sufficient to cause infection. Despite this fact, if this pandemic behaves as expected, roughly half of us will not develop symptoms of flu or if we do will have mild cases.

Diet Recommendations

Sick patients break down their muscle tissue for needed protein and calories. This is fine as long as it does not go on for long. When there is a return of appetite, this is a sign that the patient is getting better. It is important to begin feeding the patient high quality animal protein as soon as they can tolerate it to help them maintain their strength.

The Clear Liquid Diet: A clear liquid diet is used to treat certain intestinal diseases, especially infectious diarrhea. Patients suffering from diarrhea illnesses often experience abdominal

Symptom or Sign	Likely Assessment	Remedy
Low urine output	Dehydration	Push fluids
High pulse rate (>80 but especially >90)	Dehydration or fever	Push fluids
Shortness of breath	Pneumonia	Push fluids
Shaking chills/shivers	Viremia (virus in the blood) or pneumonia	Keep warm
Cyanosis (skin turns blue)	Respiratory failure that can be due to overwhelming flu pneumonia, ARDS, or secondary bacterial pneumonia. Prognosis is poor; rapid death is likely.	Keep as comfortable as possible. Give Hydrocodone with Promethazine for comfort, give diazepam for anxiety
Cough	Viral infection and irritation of the tissue lining the breathing tubes (bronchial tubes) and/or the lung tissue (alveoli) where oxygen and CO_2 are exchanged.	Push fluids, drink hot tea for effect on breathing tubes, use Hydrocodone ½ tablet with or without ½ Promethazine to suppress cough if needed
Vomiting	Virus affecting GI tract either directly or indirectly	Use Promethazine for vomiting, push fluids
Diarrhea	Virus affecting GI tract either directly or indirectly	Push ORS fluids, clear liquid diet

Symptom or Sign	Likely Assessment	Remedy
Severe stomach cramps	Virus affecting GI tract probably directly. Expect nausea, vomiting and diarrhea soon.	Use Hydrocodone and Promethazine for comfort
Bloody diarrhea but no bleeding from any other site.	This suggests the patient has the intestinal presentation of Bird flu rather than a pre-morbid development.	Use Hydrocodone and Promethazine for comfort, push ORS fluids, clear liquid diet
Headache	Due to fever	Ibuprofen and/or acetaminophen or Hydrocodone if very severe
Fever	Due to the virus stimulating the body's immune system to release chemicals that fight the infection (interferon, interleukins, cytokines)	Ibuprofen, acetaminophen, push fluids, keep warm or cool, consider tepid water baths if > 102 F. OK if <101 as this may help kill virus.
Sore throat	Direct viral infection of the posterior throat tissue. The pain is caused by inflammation or tissue breakdown there.	Gargle with hot salt water; drink hot tea or hot water, ibuprofen and or acetaminophen.
Bleeding from mouth, coughing up blood, passing red blood per rectum. Severe bruising.	A severe blood clotting abnormality has occurred due to an overwhelming flu infection (DIC). Rapid death is likely.	Keep as comfortable as possible. Give Hydrocodone with Promethazine for comfort, give diazepam for anxiety.

cramping and frequent, loose stools if they eat solid foods. In addition, a great deal of water and minerals (sodium, chloride, and potassium) are lost in the watery portion of the diarrhea stool; if you are not careful this can lead to dehydration. Patients with diarrhea have to drink considerably more fluid than usual to prevent the dehydration. This is especially important if the patient also has a fever, which in itself leads to increased loss of body water through the skin as perspiration.

In most cases, patients with diarrhea can tolerate a clear liquid diet without cramping or diarrhea. The diet starts off with clear liquids only. As symptoms abate, the diet slowly adds simple-to-digest, low-residue foods, one step at a time. Don't advance to the next step until the patient is completely symptom-free in the present step. As the patient progresses through each step, if the cramps and diarrhea return, drop back to the previous step they tolerated.

Step 1: Oral Rehydration Solution (ORS), water, fruit juice, Jell-O, Gatorade or PowerAde, ginger ale, Sprite, tea.

Step 2: Add white toast (no butter or margarine), white rice, and cream of wheat, soda crackers, and potatoes without the skin.

Step 3: To Steps 1 and 2 add canned fruit and chicken noodle soup.

Step 4: To Steps 1 through 3 add poached eggs and baked chicken breast without skin, canned fish or meat.

Step 5: To Steps 1 through 4 add milk and other dairy products, margarine or butter, raw fruits and vegetables and high-fiber whole grain products.

This same Clear Liquid Diet approach is the one to use for patients who have the flu and have been too ill to eat. They will have been on Step 1 already so when they become hungry, begin them on Step 2 and advance them through the steps as above.

Advanced Home Treatment Considerations for Health Professionals

Refer to Appendix B, page 119 for a section that discusses Tamiflu treatment and combination Probenecid with Tamiflu treatment. The section is written for healthcare professionals. It contains information that may not be wise for lay caregivers to try to use without the presence of someone who is experienced in the use of these techniques to assist you.

© Copyright by Grattan Woodson, M.D.

Adapted by the author and excerpted from the BIRD FLU PREPAREDNESS PLANNER, *with permission from the publisher: HCI Books, Deerfield, Florida*
*Available on **amazon.com**.*

→ **Preparing to Play Doctor, at a Minimum**

If there is a pandemic, prepare a sick room close to a bathroom with the supplies suggested in this chapter

---

15.
Caregiving and Grieving

Contributed by Joan Halifax, Ph.D.[1]

Support for Caregivers

Freely help those you can, but remember—
you can't help everyone.

If you're taking care of someone at home and you find yourself overwhelmed, don't feel bad. This is a normal reaction. Caregivers can, and often do, burn out because of the intense physical and emotional demands. Remember you must also take care of yourself.

You Are a Candidate for Caregiver Burnout If:

- Your hours are too long.

- You are continuously tired, irritable, or not sleeping well.

- You feel that you are caregiving alone without much support.

- You are starting to resent the patient.

    o This can evoke guilt, but guilt is pointless. You're not going to abandon a sick person because you resent them. You are probably exhausted.

- You are taking charge or making decisions without taking into consideration anyone else's feelings or opinions.

Helpful Tips for Caregivers

Self-care is the only way to build resilience.

- Set up a care-giving schedule that is sane and stick to it.

- Take breaks.

- Share responsibility and work with others as part of a team.

- Recognize the situation is not entirely in your hands.

- Get enough sleep so you can maintain perspective.

- Pace yourself.

- Take walks or get some exercise daily.

- Eat well.

- Allow yourself some quiet time just for you.

If you are a caregiver, understand you must be very careful to protect yourself while caring for the sick patient. (See Chapter 7, page 31 and Chapter 14, page 85, for more information.)

Grieving

Unexpected changes caused by any disaster can alter the course of our lives in ways that we never considered. If a loved one dies we certainly grieve; however, under the circumstances of quarantine, we also experience a sense of loss from being separated from our social and work networks. Familiar people and places are significant to our sense of identity and safety in the world. The disruption of these taken-for-granted, normal patterns of living is a loss, and with this loss comes grief.[2] Learning to grieve, to let go, to accept and finally to embrace the future takes courage and persistence.

Characteristics of Appropriate Grief

Grief is the intense emotional suffering caused by real and perceived loss. Grief is also a necessary process when events over which we have no control change our lives in ways we never expected or planned for. The following are some characteristics that support healthy grieving:[3]

- The healthy grieving process provides the opportunity for one to experience the loss and to gain insight from the experience.

- Grieving is best done in a supportive community, where interactions with others are caring and clear.

- Grief cannot be rushed. It takes time to genuinely integrate the impact of loss. Grief has no timetable.

Grief and Leave-Taking Practices

The following guidelines can assist you in working through grief:[4]

- Remember that your grief period is unique and that it involves a special awareness of your needs and feelings.

- Steps toward healing may include dream work, prayer, silent time, movement, drawing, journaling, singing, and listening to music.

- There are periods after a major change or death when a person who has suffered a loss appears in control or strong to others; however, grief is usually just below the surface and will come later.

- The expression of sadness, or even anger, is a normal part of the grieving process. Not expressing or experiencing grief increases suffering, fear, and separation.

- If someone has died, caregivers will frequently feel that they have not done enough. These feelings often can be about wishing one could have done more.

For guidelines on "Being with Dying," please refer to Appendix B, page 121.

16.
Conclusion

Now you have the information you need to prepare to survive a natural disaster, especially a bird flu pandemic. Having this knowledge doesn't mean you won't be impacted by a catastrophe. But if you have made it a priority to plan ahead to take care of yourself and the needs of your family and community, you have dramatically increased your odds of survival. Even if you never experience a major disaster, it will feel better to live in a community that has made a commitment to work together.

Everyone has an idea about how they will act in an emergency. We all want to be heroes but no one can predict what they'll do in a moment of crisis. If your car was speeding toward a cliff, you think you'd have the presence of mind to pull the emergency brake and ease onto a shoulder of the road. But unless you know what the hand brake can do and have prepared yourself mentally for this scenario, you might freeze or just grip the steering wheel and scream. Applying the information in this book helps bolster instinct with pragmatic know-how.

By the end of this book, you have taken the time to think through what you would do in a situation like a pandemic; you have the tools, supplies, and support you'll need to step up to the plate if a natural disaster occurs. During a catastrophe you'll be more resilient, less fearful, and more capable of generosity.

Share this book and these ideas with everyone in your life, near and far. Spread these ideas like a virus. The solution can be as contagious as the problem: It's up to you!

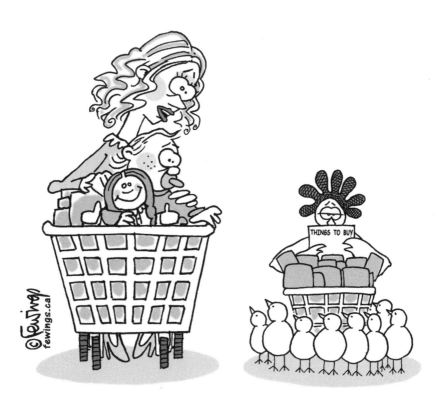

We all need to be safe if any one of us is going to be safe.

APPENDIXES A – C

→

A. Resources and References

Books

Cass, Hyla & Kathleen Barnes. *Eight Weeks to Vibrant Health.* New York: McGraw-Hill, 2004.

Davis, Mike. *The Monster at Our Door: The Global Threat of Avian Flu.* New York: The New Press, 2005.

Duhl, Leonard J. *The Urban Condition: People and Policy in the Metropolis.* New York: Basic Books, 1963.

Halifax, Joan; Barbara Dossey and Cynda Rushtin. *Compassionate Care of the Dying: An Integral Approach.* Prajna Mountain Publishers, 2005.

Siegel, Marc. *Bird Flu: Everything You Need to Know About the Next Pandemic.* Hoboken, New Jersey: John Wiley & Sons, 2006.

Woodson, Grattan. *The Bird Flu Preparadness Planner.* Deerfield Beach, Florida: Health Communications, 2005.

Articles

Brendan, Charlotte and Delay G. Hendricks. "Food Storage in the Home: Reducing Waste and Maintaining the Quality of Stored Food," Utah State University Department of Nutrition & Food Sciences, July 1995 FN 502
http://extension.usu.edu/files/foodpubs/fn502.html

Hagan, Alan. *The Prudent Pantry: Your Guide to building a Food Insurance Program.* 1999.
http://athagan.members.atlantic.net/PFSFAQ/PFSFAQ-1.html# Table%20of%20Contents

Tate, Vicki. "The Seven Major Mistakes in Food Storage," *The Preparedness Journal,* Nov/Dec 1995.
http://www.usaemergencysupply.com/information/ sevenmistakes.htm

"Growing your own food," Emergency Essential Insight Articles, Learn about growing sprouts
http://beprepared.com/article.asp?ai=66

Emergency Essentials has a series of articles about food and water storage, first aid and sanitation, and general disaster preparedness that are useful:
http://beprepared.com/article.asp_Q_ai_E_6

Websites with Information on the Avian (Bird) Flu

World Health Organization (WHO)

The WHO will track issues on a global level and report to all governments.

http://www.who.int/en

WHO Avian Influenza Frequently Asked Questions

http://www.who.int/csr/disease/avian_influenza/avian_faqs/en/
index.html#poultry

WHO Fact Sheet on Avian Influenza

http://www.who.int/csr/don/2004_01_15/en/

Centers for Disease Control and Prevention (CDC)

1-800-CDC-INFO (1-800-232-4636)

Hotline gives information on pandemic influenza. Questions can be emailed to *inquiry@cdc.gov.* The CDC will use television, radio, Internet and newspaper announcements about the status of an avian flu pandemic.

http://www.cdc.gov

Official U.S. Government Website for Information
on Pandemic Flu and Avian Influenza
http://www.pandemicflu.gov/

Review Your State's Planning Efforts
http://www.pandemicflu.gov/plan/stateplans.html

USDA Avian Influenza (Bird Flu)
*http://www.usda.gov/wps/portal/usdahome?
native=SU&navid=AVIAN_INFLUENZA*

Agricultural Department/ Animal Productive Health Division
Bird Flu and Cats.
*http://www.fao.org/ag/againfo/subjects/en/health/diseases-
cards/avian_cats.html*

Ideas For Kids In An Emergency
http://www.fema.gov/

Emergency Food & Water Supplies, FEMA
*http://www.fema.gov/areyouready/assemble_disaster_supplies_
kit.shtm*

The American Veterinary Medical Association
http://www.avma.org/

FluWiki

The purpose of the Flu Wiki is to help local communities prepare for and perhaps cope with a possible influenza pandemic.
http://www.fluwikie.com

Community Resources

Citizens Corps Programs

These programs help local citizens participate through public education and outreach, training and volunteer service through their partners: Community Emergency Response Team (CERT); Fire Corps; Neighborhood Watch (NWP); Medical Reserve Corps (MRC); Volunteers in Police Service (VIP).

https://www.citizencorps.gov/programs/

Guide to Organizing Neighborhoods for Preparedness, Response and Recovery.

The Volunteer Center of Marin, California, offers another protocol for organizing neighbors.

http://www.preparenow.org/marin-g.html

Neighborhood Watch

You may hear it called Neighborhood Watch, Home Alert, Citizen Crime Watch or Block Watch. All of the programs are neighbors working together with law enforcement to help stop a crime before it occurs. This kind of collaboration is one of the best crime-fighting teams.

http://www.nnwi.org/

Non-Violent Communication

A resource called Non Violent Communication (NVC) developed by Marshall Rosenberg, Ph.D. is a comprehensive guide to communication and conflict resolution.

http://www.cnvc.org/

Product Information

This information and more is available on the website for this book:
http://www.birdfluwhattodo.com

Water and Water Storage

55-gallon drums

http://www.quakekare.com/index.asp?PageAction=VIEWCATS
&Category=8

http://prepare411.com/food_and_water.html

Siphon pump for 55-gallon water drum
http://prepare411.com/food_and_water.html

Boxed Water Kit includes five 5-gallon Mylar water bags, 5 storage
boxes 10 tapes and instructions.
The lightproof metallized bags are spore free from the factory
to inhibit the growth of most algae and bacteria.
http://www.disasternecessities.
com/site/542519/product/KW%20S100

Reliance water storage tanks and devices
http://www.rei.com

http://www.campmor.com/webapp/wcs/stores/servlet/CategoryDi
splay?catalogId=40000000226&storeId=226&categoryId=479
24&langId=-1&parent_category_rn=252

5-Gallon Collapsible water containers
http://www.rei.com

*http://secure.lowprice4u.com:3000/Reliance-5100-15
_021080t.asp*

7-Gallon Rigid water containers
http://www.rei.com

*http://secure.lowprice4u.com:3000/Reliance-8930-03
_016876t.asp*

Potable Agua has an iodine tablet treatment where one tablet neutralizes the taste of iodine. Lemon is another way of neutralizing the taste.
http://www.rei.com

*http://www.shopzilla.com/8B--Camping_Hiking_Gear_-
_SEARCH_GO--Find%20it!__cat_id--12040100__keyword--
aqua%20iodine%20tablet__search_box--1__sfsk--1*

First Need Delux Water Purifier made by General Ecology is a purifier that has a 125 gallon capacity, and is what I have purchased.
http://www.rei.com

Strepin has a purifier that uses an ultra violet treatment method. Systems that use a ceramic filter require cleaning and maintenance. All are available at R.E.I.
http://www.rei.com

Long-term water disinfection and storage information
http://www.storablefoods.com/water_storage.html

Food and Food Storage

General Information
> *http://waltonfeed.com/self/seven.html*

Information about solar cooking
> *http://www.solarcooking.org/*

Emergency Food
> *http://www.nitvo-pad.com/*

Sanitation Supplies

SaniDex Antimicrobial Wipes
> *http://prepare411.com/first_aid_and_trauma_supplies.html*

A recommended N95 mask called NanoMask
> *http://www.buynanomask.com*

Alcohol based sanitizers and Antimicrobial products such as AprilGuard Antiseptic Handrub or Avant Original
> *http://www.sanitationtools.com/Products.*
> *asp?Product=1416&Category=9*

> *http://www.Alwaysbeprepared.com*

> *http://www.alwaysbeprepared.com/site/558697/page/150887*

Bio Gel Waste Gelatin:
> a sewage chemical treatment pack for disinfecting human waste
> *http://secure.lowprice4u.com:3000/Reliance-2681-13_016936t.asp*

Power Supplies

Shut off wrench for utilities

http://secure.lowprice4u.com:3000/Reliance-2681-13_016936t.asp

Liquid Paraffin candles, alternative to candles, are smokeless and good for indoors.

http://glassdimensions.com/s.nl/sc.9/.f

http://www.discountcandleshop.com/product_info. php/products_id/2294

http://candles.genwax.com/candle_groups/___0___lamp_oil.htm

Gerber makes a long distance L.E.D. with intense light.

http://www.rei.com

Nightstar CS Flashlight generates energy as you move it. Cost approximately $30.

http://www.rei.com

Propane stoves and canisters

http://www.rei.com

Esbit Pocket Stove is an emergency stove used by the military that costs about $10.00. It's a short-term solution, the heat source is a tablet, and so you would need a stock of tablets.

http://www.rei.com

Nuwick candles and their folding stove

http.://www.campmor.com

http://www.nitro-pak.com

General Camping and Emergency Supplies

Camping Supplies

http://www.rei.com

http://www.campmor.com

A good hand cranked radio: Eton

http://www.rei.com

http://www.amazon.com

B. Additional Health Considerations

1. Patient Prognosis During Pandemic Influenza

Excerpted from "Good Home Care For Patients With Bird Flu" by Grattan Woodson, M.D., F.A.C.P.

One thing that is different about a major pandemic is just how hard it hits patients and how rapidly it kills. Patients affected by the flu can be categorized broadly into 3 prognostic types. The first type has a poor prognosis no matter what is done for them. The second might survive if there was full access to high technology medical care and resources. The third type is highly likely to recover from the flu as long as they are provided with consistent low-technology supportive measures that can be administered in home settings.

Type 1 patients have the poorest prognosis and almost all will die within 2 or 3 days of the development of their first symptoms. The cause of death in these patients during the 1918 flu was massive respiratory failure from overwhelming lung-destroying viral pneumonia. There was no effective treatment for this in 1918, and there is none today despite all the advances in medicine that have occurred over the last 90 years. Signs and symptoms of type 1 patients include rapid onset of severe shortness of breath, cyanosis (bluish discoloration of the skin of the hands, feet, and around the mouth and spreading centrally), or bleeding from the lungs, stomach and rectum.

Type 2 patients are similar to type 1 patients except they do not die after 3 days. Some but not many of these patients would survive if they had access to an ICU, ventilators and expert medical care but if we have a severe pandemic, those resources will not be widely available. Even if they had access to these services, many of them would die anyway. Remember, no matter what you do, they are likely to pass away in a week to 10 days after becoming ill.

Type 3 patients make up the majority of those that become ill with influenza. Fortunately, these patients have a good prognosis if they receive timely and diligent supportive care that can be provided well in a non-medical setting such as the home. Most of these pandemic flu victims will be so severely ill and weakened by the infection that they will be too ill to get out of bed. Many type 3 patients will be completely dependent on others for care. Without simple care, some of these patients will die from preventable causes like dehydration, but with simple care, most of these patients will recover. No matter how good the care provided, some type 3 patients will die. This is not your fault. This happens usually because they develop a serious secondary condition that actually becomes the cause of death. Examples of these secondary conditions include bacterial pneumonia, stroke, and heart attack. There is nothing you can do but keep doing the best you can and let nature take its course.

In my opinion, as a general rule, provide everyone with the same level of supportive care. This is a rational course because it is not always possible to predict who will survive and who will not, especially early in the course of the flu.

2. Advanced Home Treatment Considerations for Healthcare Professionals

Excerpted from "Good Home Care for Patients with Bird Flu" by Grattan Woodson, M.D.

The section is written for healthcare professionals. It contains information that may not be wise for lay caregivers to use without the presence of someone who is experienced in the use of these techniques to assist you.

Tamiflu Treatment

If you have access to Tamiflu, the dose is one tablet twice daily for 5 days. It is best to begin Tamiflu within two days of the beginning of symptoms but might be useful when used even later in the course. I recommend using Tamiflu even if there are widespread reports of Tamiflu resistance in the strains circulating in your area. The reason has to do with the fact that for the bird flu to become resistant, there must be a mutation that makes it less virulent. So, the patient still gets sick but with a strain that is less likely to kill.

Combination of Probenecid with Tamiflu

Use of Probenecid 500 mg twice daily during Tamiflu administration increases the plasma level of Tamiflu by 2 times and the half-life by 2.5 times. This means that you can significantly extend the supply of this crucial antiviral agent if you have it available to you. This strategy is safe as the therapeutic index of Tamiflu is quite wide and the side effects of the two drugs are minor. Probenecid blocks renal tubular secretion of Tamiflu reducing its excretion in the urine by 60%. It has a similar effect on -lactam class antibiotics and all NSAIDs. The doses of these other products need to be reduced when given with Probenecid.

© Copyright by Grattan Woodson, M.D.

Appendixes 1 and 2 are adapted by the author and excerpted from the BIRD FLU PREPAREDNESS PLANNER, *with permission from the publisher: HCI Books, Deerfield, Florida. Available on* ***amazon.com.***

3. End-of-Life Decisions

Contributed by Joan Halifax, Ph.D.

People often have preferences about how they want to die.

- Who will make healthcare decisions when they can't?
- What kind of medical treatment do they want?
- How comfortable or pain-free do they want to be?
- What information do they want their support team to have?

Advance Medical Directives[1]

Two common types of advance medical directives are:

- Living Wills
- Durable Power of Attorney for Health Care.

A Living Will is a document in which a person can give instructions about their health care if, in the future, they cannot communicate or make decisions. This includes the kind of health care a person does or does not want. Such a directive only becomes relevant when the person no longer has the capacity to make his or her own decisions.

A *Durable Power of Attorney for Health Care* allows a person to name someone to be their representative, sometimes called an agent or proxy, to make health care decisions when they can no longer speak for themselves. Increasingly, patients and families are advised to designate a person for this role in advance of serious illness and to discuss preferences for treatment and end-of-life decisions. Without the designation of a proxy, state laws governing designation of decision-makers would apply. This is particularly important for patients who would not choose to have traditional decision-makers such as spouses, parents, children, etc. appointed to speak on their behalf.

Informed Consent is a process to assure that patients or their surrogates are fully informed of relevant information so that they can make a voluntary choice about treatment options.

4. Being with Dying
Contributed by Joan Halifax, Ph.D.

For many of us, being with someone who is critically ill or facing death is unknown territory. It will be challenging, to say the least. Just know there is no right way to be and that simply being there is the most important thing. Even if someone is in a coma, never underestimate the value of touch and the impact of your presence.

Extremely ill or dying people are for the most part justifiably self-preoccupied and can easily feel confused by the overwhelming experience. They can be absorbed in their pain and experience of being sick.

Treat a critically ill or dying person with respect. Stay physically and psychologically attentive to the person you are caring for:

- Ask them what they want and need rather than assuming you know.
- Offer them control over those things that they want to manage.
- Actively encourage them to do what they want for as long as they can, whether it be walking to the toilet or making decisions about what to eat or with whom to visit.
- Accept and appreciate silences rather than feeling the need for constant talk. There is no need to divert or entertain a person who is ill or dying.
- Sit with the person and reminisce.
- Give them sponge baths.
- Tend to your grief away from persons you are taking care of.
- Give advice only when asked.
- Offer repeated assurances that you can help them with their symptoms.
- Tell them to not worry about incontinence.

A Supportive Environment

You can create a supportive, calm environment for those who are very ill or dying. Reassure the critically ill or dying person that you are with them. If, or when, the final moments before death come, keep the atmosphere around the dying person calm and quiet.

Immediately After Death

- Continue to keep the atmosphere around the deceased simple and peaceful.
- Creating rituals to mark the passing of a life can be healing to family members and to health care professionals. Simple acts such as a moment of silence can signify reverence and respect.
- Methods of caring for the body of the deceased vary from culture to culture, and these customs should be respected if possible.

Appendixes 3 and 4 adapted by the author from
Compassionate Care of the Dying: An Integral
Approach *by Joan Halifax, Barbara Dossey, and Cynda
Rushtin, with permission from Prajna Mountain Publishers.*

5. If Someone Dies at Home

Knowing what bodily changes to expect when someone dies will help lessen the fear and shock at the moment of death. In the case of the bird flu, it is likely these changes will be seen as death approaches: Choking on secretion, cyanosis (skin turns blue or dusky), shortness of breath, a heart rate over 150, and sweating. If the person goes into shock, which may happen shortly before they die, you will notice cold extremities and an elevated and weak pulse. If you have concerns about how to comfort someone who is very ill or dying, ask your local health officials for additional suggestions.

Several physicians have advised me that people who are dying from influenza have a sense of drowning and that opiates alleviate this sensation. If you are taking care of a dying person, contact hospice or a doctor who will prescribe appropriate medications to ease an end-of-life situation. Also ask your local public health officials what measures would be taken to ease end-of-life suffering in a bird flu pandemic if health facilities were overwhelmed.

If many public systems are overwhelmed and there is a death at home, you need to find out what procedures to follow. Call your local health officials, local police, and fire departments and get this information from them now. If they have not thought through these issues, encourage them to do so before there is an emergency situation such as a pandemic, where ordinary procedures in caring for the deceased might be interrupted.

How to Handle a Body After Death Has Occurred

Call the coroner's office during a natural disaster after a death at home. If is functioning, they will come and remove the body. Body handling should be left to trained medical staff designated by the coroner's office. If this is not possible because of a breakdown of infrastructure, attending to the body immediately after death is important.

- When touching the body use protective gloves and a N95 mask if the person has died of the bird flu.
- Fluid-proof Vinyl or Latex gloves should be worn.[3]
  o These should be disposed of with other sickroom waste.

- Hands and other skin surfaces should be washed immediately and thoroughly if contaminated with blood or other body fluids and after gloves are removed.
- Use a chlorine sanitizing solution for disinfectant.
- At the point of death the dying person may have defecated, urinated, or vomited.
- Be careful with all waste materials, as they may be contagious.
- The body needs to stay as cool as possible if there is a chance it will be picked up within a few days. A fan, air conditioning, dry ice, or an open window can be helpful in keeping the body fresh.
- Body bags will further reduce the risk of infection.

What to Do with the Body

In the United States, a doctor needs to sign a death certificate. It isn't necessary that the doctor come to the deceased. In ordinary circumstances when you contact the coroner's office, a crematorium or a burial society, they come within a short period of time.

Burial is the preferred method of body disposal in emergency situations unless there are cultural or religious observances that prohibit it. Burial on your own property is permitted in many places in the United States. If home burial is chosen, keep in mind that future owners of the land may move the grave or may not permit it to be visited.

- In a pandemic, burial or cremations should take place soon after death at a site near the place of death.

- Burial procedures should be consistent with the usual practices of the community concerned.
- The location of graveyards should be agreed upon with the community and attention should be given to ground conditions, proximity to groundwater drinking sources, and to the nearest habitation.
- Burial in individual graves, dug manually, is preferred.
- If health officials cannot remove the body of the deceased and it cannot be stored in a safe place, it should be buried.
- In an emergency, if you have a yard, bury the deceased in your yard.
- If coffins are not available, corpses should be wrapped in plastic sheeting to keep the remains separate from the soil.[2]
  - o Before covering a corpse with dirt, it is helpful to place branches, wire mesh, or some barrier over the corpse, followed by the soil. In this way, dogs, or other animals, will be discouraged from digging and uncovering the corpse.[3]

For emotional and psychological reasons, be sure to be able to identify the body by clearly marking the body's wrapping, tying an identity tag to the body, and marking the burial site. The identification should include the legal name, date of birth, gender, date of death, and circumstance of death.

If you must take charge of the burial of a body, protect yourself as much as possible. You are still here and your survival is important.

C. Master Lists

1: The Top Twenty

1. A plan with your neighborhood
2. Baking soda or lime carbonate
3. Battery operated or hand-cranked radio
4. Bleach for water purification and sanitation purposes
5. Chocolate, or comfort food
6. Extra prescription medications
7. Flashlights and batteries
8. Food supplies for at least 30 days per person
9. Gloves, both surgical and work
10. Heavy duty garbage bags and duct tape
11. Home pharmacy items such as table salt, sugar and baking soda
12. Liquid soap, antiseptic hand wash
13. N95 masks
14. Neighborhood contact list
15. Paper towels
16. Some form of aspirin (e.g. some form of ibuprofen)
17. Stove and fuel for cooking
18. Toilet paper
19. Water containers to store water for 30 days per person (e.g. 60 gallons)
20. Wrenches to turn off water and gas utilities

2: Food Storage Supplies

Freeze-Dried or Dehydrated Foods

Consider buying #10 cans of freeze-dried or dehydrated foods instead of canned food. A #10 can holds more freeze-dried food than regular food. They have a shelf life of 5 years, longer than the 1 year for regular canned foods.

Staples You Might Already Have

- Salt
- Pepper
- Baking powder
- Baking soda
- Spices
- Sugar
- Honey
- Flour
- Vanilla Extract
- Oil, canola or olive
- Chocolate
- Tea
- Coffee
- Low sodium bouillon
- Dry soup mixes
- Vinegar

Fresh Foods That Store More Easily

These can be kept up to a few months if stored in a cool dry place.

- Onions
- Garlic
- Potatoes
- Sweet potatoes
- Yams
- Beets
- Turnips
- Chili peppers
- Carrots
- Sprouts
- Lemons
- Apples, fresh or dried

Canned Goods or Goods in Jars
- ❑ Tuna fish, sardines, salmon
- ❑ Peanut butter
- ❑ Jams
- ❑ Juices
- ❑ Soy or rice milk
- ❑ Evaporated Milk
- ❑ Drinks with electrolytes such as Gatorade
- ❑ Pet Food (both dried & canned)
- ❑ Baby food (if applicable

Dried Food
- ❑ Onions
- ❑ Peas
- ❑ Jerky
- ❑ Rice
- ❑ Cereals
- ❑ Crackers
- ❑ Powdered drink mixes
- ❑ Dried fruits
- ❑ Lentils
- ❑ Beans
- ❑ Milk - powdered
- ❑ Pasta
- ❑ Oatmeal
- ❑ Ovaltine
- ❑ Nuts
- ❑ Dried meals
- ❑ High-energy bars such as Granola, Power Bars, etc.

3: Home Supplies

- ❑ Water containers (See Chapter 2, page 8.)
- ❑ Food containers (food grade only—check this with your hardware store)
- ❑ Washboard
- ❑ Home use chlorine such as Clorox
- ❑ Purification tablets or iodine
- ❑ Alcohol
- ❑ Hand operated can opener—buy two as gears easily strip
- ❑ Gas & water wrench
- ❑ Clothespins and line
- ❑ Liquid laundry detergent
- ❑ Paper plates
- ❑ Plastic utensils
- ❑ Paper towels
- ❑ Aluminum foil
- ❑ Ziplock bags for storing food
- ❑ Antibacterial soap
- ❑ Duct tape
- ❑ Scissors
- ❑ Saw
- ❑ Hammer
- ❑ Screwdriver
- ❑ Shovel
- ❑ Wheelbarrow or pull cart
- ❑ Work gloves
- ❑ Clothes for winter weather
- ❑ Baby supplies including diapers, baby food, and formula
- ❑ Pet supplies (if applicable)

4: Hygiene and Home Pharmacy Supplies

❑ Toilet paper

❑ Alcohol hand disinfectants

❑ Antiseptic soap

❑ Antiseptic Toilettes

❑ Antimicrobial Wipes

❑ Alcohol

❑ Hydrogen peroxide

❑ Soap bars

❑ Shampoo

❑ Heavy-duty plastics garbage bags or Plastic sheeting

❑ Toothbrushes

❑ Toothpaste

❑ Feminine hygiene products

❑ Razor blades

❑ Shaving cream

❑ Extra prescription medications

❑ Basic first aid kit with bandages, etc.

❑ Thermometers - at least two

❑ Pain medication: Aspirin, Ibuprofen, Tylenol

❑ Antacid

❑ Medication for diarrhea

❑ Contact lenses solution if needed

❑ Protective surgical gloves

❑ N95 masks

5: Preparing for a Power Outage

❑ Matches: books, boxes. Do not store all matches in one place.

❑ Candles, preferably long-lasting ones.

❑ Liquid paraffin (an alternative to candles) is smokeless and safe for indoors.

❑ Extra batteries: back up quantities for all battery operated devices you have.

❑ Oil & wicks for lanterns if needed.

❑ Extra fuses (for old fashioned electrical systems).

❑ L.E.D flashlights are not expensive and last longer than flashlights that use regular batteries.

❑ L.E.D. flashlight that fits on your head. Petzl has one that last 150 hours at low setting, 80 hours at a high setting.

❑ Long distance L.E.D. flashlight.

❑ Hand-generated flashlight.

❑ Battery charger: solar powered or with a hand-crank.

❑ Propane canisters/kerosene that matches your equipment.

❑ Hand-cranked or battery-operated radio.

❑ Solar-powered calculator.

❑ Gasoline generators are an expensive but possible option.

6: Cooking without Power

❏ Outdoor barbecue grill
❏ Extra briquettes
❏ Propane tank(s) for outdoor grill
❏ Coleman stove using propane canisters
❏ Esbit Pocket Stove (See page 21, "Cooking without Power" for a more detail description of this)
❏ Trangia Minitrangia 28-T Stove uses denatured (drug store) alcohol as a heat source.
❏ Nuwick candles and their folding stove
❏ Extra tanks and canisters for your cooking device

7: Useful Solar-Powered Items

❏ 3-in-1 socket multiplier (transforms car cigarette lighter) Turns into three 12 volt outlets for use with TVs, power inverters, boom-boxes, cellular phones, power tools, lamps, car vacuums, etc.)
❏ 13 watt solar charger (used to power hand tools, DC refrigerator, laptop computer, DPS systems, etc.)
❏ Solar-powered battery charger
❏ Solar-powered calculator
❏ Solar phone charger
❏ Solar-powered refrigerator
❏ Solar-powered electric vehicles Power Generation System (The EN-R-PAK model by BA Products weighs 80 pounds, is portable and quiet, doesn't emit exhaust fumes, and provides approx. 20 hours of usage when fully charged)
❏ Solar/crank Radio
❏ Solar/crank Flashlight and Lantern

8: Combating Boredom: Entertaining Ideas

❑ Board games   ❑ Playing cards

❑ Books to read   ❑ Songbooks

❑ Dice   ❑ Puzzles, etc.

❑ Radio: battery-operated with plenty of batteries

❑ Instruments to play

❑ Simple exercise or sports equipment
    (depending on the region and season)

9: Keeping Your ID[4]

❑ Driver's License   ❑ Passport/Green Card

❑ Birth Certificate   ❑ Power(s) of Attorney

❑ Marriage License   ❑ Divorce Papers

❑ Social Security Card

❑ Naturalization Documents

Personal Property

❑ Mortgage or Real Estate Deeds of Trust

❑ Vehicle Registration/Ownership Papers

Tax Statements

❑ Previous Year's Tax Returns

❑ Property Tax Statement

Latest Statement of Financial Accounts

❑ Bank/Credit Union Statements

❑ Credit/Debit Card Statements

❑ Retirement Accounts (401K, TSP, IRA)

❑ Investment Accounts (Stocks, Bonds, Mutual Funds)

Information for Sources of Income/Assets

☐ Government Benefits (e.g. Social Security, Temporary
  Assistance for Needy Families)
☐ Alimony Income
☐ Child Support Income
☐ Professional Appraisals of Personal Property
☐ Rewards Accounts (e.g., Frequent Flyer, Hotel Rewards)

Financial Obligations Information

☐ Mortgage Statement ☐ Car Payment
☐ Student Loan ☐ Alimony Payments
☐ Child Support Payments ☐ Other Debt
☐ Utility Bills (Gas/Electric, Water)

Insurance Information

☐ Property Insurance ☐ Rental Insurance
☐ Auto Insurance ☐ Life Insurance

Medical Information

☐ Health Insurance ID Card(s)
☐ Record of Immunizations/Allergies
☐ List of Necessary Medications
☐ Disability Documents ☐ Living Will
☐ Dental Records ☐ Child Identity Cards
☐ Durable Power of Attorney

Military Records

☐ Current Military ID
☐ Military Discharge DD 2

Notes

CHAPTER 2

1. Managing Water Supplies. FEMA.
   http://www.fema.gov/plan/prepare/watermanage.shtm

2. *http://www.thefarm.org/charities/i4at/surv/bleach.htm*

3. *http://www.fema.gov/pdf/library/f&web.pdf*

4. This water is not safe for drinking as there will probably be some bacteria in it from people's bodies, in addition to body oils, pollution from the air, etc. Also, chemicals used in swimming pools and spas are too concentrated for safe drinking. This water can be used for cleaning and related uses.
   http://www.fema.gov/plan/prepare/watermanage.shtm

CHAPTER 3

1. *http://www.cfsan.fda.gov/~dms/avfluqa.html*

CHAPTER 4

1. Pure denatured alcohol. Denatured alcohol can be dissolved in water for cleaning. Can also be used in alcohol type stoves. The "denatured" in its name refers to the fact that chemicals have been added so this alcohol is toxic or distasteful, and should not be consumed. It is still useful as a household chemical.
   http://www.wikipedia.org/wiki/denatured_alcohol

CHAPTER 7

1. No mask can provide a perfect barrier; but products that meet or exceed the NIOSH 95 (N95) standard recommended by the World Health Organization and Centers for Disease Control are thought to provide good protection. A N95 mask (actually called a respirator) is a personal protective device that is worn on the face, covers at least the nose and mouth, and is used to reduce the wearer's risk of inhaling hazardous airborne particles including dust particles and infectious agents, gases, or vapors. The CDC recommends that health care workers protect themselves

from any disease spread through the air (airborne transmission) by wearing a respirator at least as protective as a fit-tested N95 mask.
http://www.cdc.gov/niosh/npptl/topics/respirators/factsheets/ respsars.html

2. Contributed by Hyla Cass, M.D., whose website has information on integrative medicine and resources on alternative medicine. *http://www.cassmd*

CHAPTER 9

1. U.S. Senate Majority Leader Bill Frist's keynote address to the National Press Club on December 8, 2005.
http://frist.senate.gov/index.cfm?FuseAction=Speeches. Detail&Speech_id=322&Month=12&Year=2005

2. This is the service that emergency management consultants like the author of this section provides for organizations.

CHAPTER 13

1. This brochure was developed and produced by a group of health care professionals who obtained a grant from the American Red Cross Northern California Disaster Preparedness Network. The group works in San Jose, California, for Good Samaritan Hospital and the Planetree Health Library. The American Red Cross Disaster Education Program helps people avoid, prepare for, and cope with disasters that may occur. To obtain hard copies of this brochure, write to Planetree Health Library, Mission Oaks campus, 15891 Los Gatos-Almaden Road, Los Gatos, CA 95032, or contact *www.planetreesanjose.org.*

2. Researchers at Erasmus Medical Center have demonstrated systemic spread of avian influenza virus in cats infected by respiratory, digestive, and cat-to-cat contact. The paper by Rimmelzwaan et.al., "Influenza A virus (H5N1) infection in cats causes systemic disease with potential novel routes of virus spread within and between hosts," appears in the January 2006 issue of *The American Journal of Pathology.*

CHAPTER 14

1. Tamiflu is expensive, costing about $200 for 20 tablets. If you have insurance, you will still pay a significant co-pay. All the other prescription drugs are generic and not expensive.

2. The color, sediment, and feel of urine can all be of help in determining dehydration. Dark urine with lots of sediment that feels thick between your fingers is very likely to be highly concentrated indicating that the patient is dehydrated and needs more ORS.

CHAPTER 15

1. Adapted by the author from *Compassionate Care of the Dying: An Integral Approach* by Joan Halifax, Barbara Dossey, and Cynda Rushtin, with permission from Prajna Mountain Publishers.

2. Fried, Marc. "Grieving for a Lost Home." *The Urban Condition: People and Policy in the Metropolis.* Ed.Leonard J. Duhl. New York: Basic Books, 1963. 151-171.

3. Based on the work of David Feinstein and Mayo, 1990.

4. Based on Olsen and Dossey, 2005.

APPENDICES

1. Aging with Dignity is a non-profit that provides advice and legal tools for elders to ensure their final wishes are respected. *http://www.agingwithdignity.org/*

2. World Health Organization, "Disposal of dead bodies in emergency conditions." *http://wedc.lboro.ac.uk/WHO_Technical _Notes_for_Emergencies/8%20-%20Disposal%20of%20dead% 20bodies.pdf*

3. Eduardo Furher Jiménez, veterinarian with the Servicio Agrícola y Ganadero del Ministerio de Agricultura de Chile (Agriculture and Livestock Service of the Ministry of Agriculture of Chile). *http://www.crid.or.cr/digitalizacion/pdf/eng/doc15631/ doc15631.pdf*

4. This list is adapted from the Emergency Financial First Aid Kit © sponsored by Operation HOPE, Inc, FEMA, Citizen's Corp.

Author and Contributors

Verona Fonté, Ph.D., author of *Bird Flu What To Do,* worked as a psychologist for over twenty years in academic, clinical and organizational settings. She was Academic Dean at the Saybrook Institute serving a faculty comprised of the founders of Humanistic Psychology such as Rollo May, Jim Bugenthal and Stanley Krippner. In her professional capacity, Dr. Fonté was at the forefront of the initial programs that emerged into the managed health care model of the early 1980's. For twelve years she served as a member of a trauma team within a division of the Department of Justice. Currently she is on the Board of Directors of Peaceworkers International and is an advocate of non-violence. She has worked with children of war and youth leaders from war-torn areas in many capacities.

In 1994, while on a work trip to Dagestan, a region of the former Soviet Union surrounded by Chechnya, Georgia and Azerbaijan, Dr. Fonté heard a story that changed her life. A young Russian filmmaker recording the trip told her he had refused to go into the Russian military. The KGB persuaded his mother to sign him into a mental hospital where he spent 2 years on medications he knew nothing about, not knowing if he would ever get out. On hearing this story, Dr. Fonté decided she could no longer listen to people's stories that had to be held in confidence for professional reasons. At that point in her life, to become part of the group that helped get stories out into the world, she became a filmmaker and director of the public charity, Iris Arts & Education Group, which has a mission to produce and support socially relevant media, educational and artistic products.

Dr. Fonté's first short documentary, "The Peaceful Warrior," is about what she found in Dagestan in the mid-nineties. In 2001, she made another short documentary, "Quest For Justice," about Soon Duk Kim, a former Korean "comfort woman." The film uses artwork made by Kim and other former comfort women to tell the story of sexual slavery by the Japanese military in World War II.

A similar life-changing moment occurred when Dr. Fonté's friend, Dr. Ted Mohns, told her a story in December 2005 that reflected the reality that many people will be on their own if there is a global pandemic. Compelled to action by a need to do something useful to help this situation, and inspired by a conversation with another close friend, Dan Smith, about the altruism that emerged during the great plague in London in the 17th century, Dr. Fonté took on the assignment of writing this book. *Bird Flu What to Do: Prepare to Survive* is a product of her sense of urgency about preparing for natural disasters and her steadfast belief that people must work together in their preparations for survival.

Dr. Fonté lives in Berkeley, California and can be reached at *verona@veronafonte.com*

Visit the website for *Bird Flu What to Do: Prepare to Survive*
www.birdfluwhattodo.com

CONTRIBUTORS

Grattan Woodson, M.D., F.A.C.P. obtained his M.D. at the Medical College of Georgia in 1980 and completed a categorical internal medicine residency training at The Mary Imogene Bassett Hospital in Cooperstown, N.Y., an affiliate of Columbia University College of Physicians and Surgeons in New York, N.Y. In 1983, Dr. Woodson joined the full-time faculty of Emory University School of Medicine where he began his work in osteoporosis. In 1986 he left Emory to form the Osteoporosis Center of Atlanta, where he focused his efforts on the diagnosis and treatment of patients with osteoporosis, osteoporosis research, and physician education. He is the also the author of a number of articles on the diagnosis and treatment of this disease. He remains active in physician education and maintains his relationship with Emory University where he serves as a Clinical Instructor of Medicine.

Edward B. (Ted) Mohns, M.D. of Del Mar, CA, provides consulting services to biotechnology and technology companies, and has consulted to a venture capital group in addition to his own angel investment activities. Trained in Internal Medicine at Stanford and in Psychiatry at UCSD, Dr. Mohns maintains a part-time clinical practice, is Associate Clinical Professor, UCSD School of Medicine, is involved in the therapeutic applications of low-energy laser, and has long been active in medical ethics. He also serves on the board of the Verified Voting Foundation as well as pursuing a variety of other civic interests. Dr. Mohns first became alerted to avian flu in 2004, and since then has been working intently on this issue at multiple levels.

Joshua D. Lichterman, Ph.D. is the owner and President of the Emergency Management Group Inc. of Grass Valley, CA. He has been a Business Continuity Planner for more than 27 years and has worked with a variety of clients in both the public and private sectors. He has performed risk assessments and vulnerability analyses, developed business continuity plans, and developed and delivered related training and exercise programs. He taught at the California Specialized Training Institute and the UC Berkeley Extension Certificate Program in Emergency Management. His clients have included Neutrogena Corp., Chevron, Berkeley Unified School District, City of Berkeley, California Department of Rehabilitation, and Genentech Corp. His email address is *joshemgi@mac.com*

Kathleen Johnson, M.S., R.D, received degrees in nutrition from the University of Arizona. She has been working as a nutritionist for over 25 years, beginning in public health nutrition and nutrition education and moving toward her interest in preventive nutrition and the education of health professionals and the public. She worked 12 years at Canyon Ranch Health Resort and 3 years as the nutritionist with Dr. Andrew Weil's Program in Integrative Medicine at the University of Arizona. She is now a consulting nutritionist with National University and Canyon Ranch.

Joan Halifax, Ph.D., is an anthropologist, social activist, and Buddhist teacher. She founded the Ojai Foundation, The Upaya Zen Center, the Project on Being with Dying, and the Upaya Prison Project. She was on the faculty to Columbia University, the New School for Social Research, and Naropa University. She was an Honorary Research Fellow at Harvard University, received a National Science Foundation Fellowship, and is the author of numerous books, including "Compassionate Care of the Dying: An Integral Approach." She is Abbot of Upaya Zen Center, and teaches world wide on the subject of death and dying. She is also Verona Fonté's sister.